BULLETIN 344

Women coping with HIV/AIDS

We take it as it is

JUDITH VAN WOUDENBERG

ROYAL TROPICAL INSTITUTE - AMSTERDAM

Bulletins of the Royal Tropical Institute

The Bulletin series of the Royal Tropical Institute (KIT) deals with current themes in international development cooperation. KIT Bulletins offer a multi-disciplinary forum for scientists and development workers active in agricultural and enterprise development; health; and culture, history and anthropology. These fields reflect the broad scope of Royal Tropical Institute activities.

Bulletins can be ordered separately or on a standing order: an invoice will be sent with each publication.

Information

Royal Tropical Institute
KIT Press
P.O. Box 95001
1090 HA Amsterdam
The Netherlands
Telephone: 31 (20) 5688272
Telefax: 31 (20) 5688286
E-mail: kitpress@kit.nl
Website: http://www.kit.nl

Publications

We would like to thank the AIDS Counselling Trust (ACT) for permission to use their poster 'Care enough to love safely' on the cover. The ACT is not, however, the anonymous organization referred to in this Bulletin.

The phrase 'We take it as it is' in the title is a translation of the Shona saying 'Tave kuzvigamuchira sezvazviri'

Author's dedication:
This publication is dedicated to my 'sister' Beauty (Tsitsi in this book), who died on January 2nd 1994, after a long period of illness.

© 1998 – Royal Tropical Institute
Cover: Nel Punt – Amsterdam
Illustration front cover: AIDS Counselling Trust (ACT), Harare, Zimbabwe
Printing: Ars Nova, Hendrik Ido Ambacht
ISBN 90 6832 8344
NUGI 661

Table of contents

Summary

This Bulletin is based on a 14 month medical anthropological study of the consequences of HIV and AIDS for HIV-positive women in Zimbabwe, their coping strategies and the support they needed and received. The qualitative study took place within Sikukuchwa,[1] an organization in Harare which supports people, and women in particular, who have HIV or AIDS. Field work was conducted in April – July 1993, when 19 of the 35 women participating at Sikukuchwa were interviewed in depth.

HIV/AIDS appeared to be the object of stigmatization. All Sikukuchwa participants were reluctant to reveal their HIV status to relatives, close friends or others in their community. Rejection or abandonment, however, rarely occurred. The fear of stigma was greater than that justified by the reality. Nevertheless, it was noticeable that these women did not talk even with people they met outside Sikukuchwa whom they presumed to be HIV positive, although many stated they would like to help those people. HIV infection within a marital or non-marital relationship was a particularly sensitive issue. Seven of 19 relationships had broken up directly or indirectly due to HIV. The women's socioeconomic conditions had also changed considerably since their diagnosis as HIV positive. HIV/AIDS drained their resources and their living standards decreased. One of the greatest psychological consequences for HIV-positive women was uncertainty about the future; recurring symptoms were constant reminders of their disease. Some women expressed fears concerning their own well being, and most were worried about their children's future.

Women at Sikukuchwa made use of various coping strategies. Their coping was often emotion focused (religion, positive reinterpretation, acceptance, seeking emotional social support, and/or denial). Further, they turned to some types of problem-focused coping (active coping and planning) and two other coping responses, mental disengagement and hope. Coping appeared to occur in stages, roughly following the progression from HIV infection to full-blown AIDS. The value of the Sikukuchwa project was that it helped HIV-positive women develop coping strategies, emotionally and (through income-generating activities) economically. Most women realized they were not passive victims of this disease and that they could do something about their situation themselves, for example by caring for their health and living positively within the group of women participating in the project. However, at Sikukuchwa the focus of coping was on the individual. On the one hand Sikukuchwa supported HIV-positive women greatly and created a safe environment. On the other hand, as a consequence the project to some extent impeded coping as a part of normal life; for example, it did not stimulate women to reveal their HIV status in their own environments or to assist others with the same problem.

Acknowledgements

As a student in medical biology, I experienced the strengths of the discipline as well as its limitations. Whereas much attention was paid to the medical side of diseases and health and to epidemiology, social aspects of illness were virtually ignored. I gradually became aware that illness is thoroughly interwoven with social, cultural and emotional aspects. With respect to sexually related diseases and sexual behaviour, for example, people often do not practise what they say is right, or what they seem to want. This area is full of taboos, morals, emotions and fears. AIDS as a new disease confronts and challenges people with dilemmas. It brings up many complexities and extremities of life: illness, sexual relationships, choice, behavioural change and threats of divorce, poverty and death.

In the course on health education and prevention in the Department of Biological Education, University of Utrecht, I met Dr. Arend Jan Waarlo and Prof. Peter Voogt. Both were very stimulating and encouraged me to choose this unusual path to complete my studies in biology. My first practical experience in health education was with the Dutch STD Foundation. There I was confronted with STD/AIDS prevention and health promotion. Gradually my involvement with people who had HIV/AIDS became more intense. As awareness of the AIDS explosion in Africa increased I wanted to understand the African context better. For that reason my next stop was the Department of Medical Anthropology at the University of Amsterdam, where I met Prof. Sjaak van der Geest. I am very grateful to him for bringing me into contact with Prof. Corlien Varkevisser, also attached to the Department of Medical Anthropology and to the Royal Tropical Institute. Under her guidance I carried out the research project described here at Sikukuchwa, a centre for HIV-positive women in Harare, Zimbabwe.

This study dealt with the most intimate subjects of sexuality and death. Therefore, I asked my informants whether they would allow me to interview them and ultimately to publish the results. They had no objections to publication as long as it was not in Zimbabwe. They wanted to keep their HIV-status a secret, for fear of stigmatization, rejection and discrimination. This is highly understandable. Hence I have changed their names as well as that of the organization. Sikukuchwa, the Kiswahili name used here for the organization, means 'the dawn of a new life', something the organization stands for. The women's names have been inspired by people I met in Zimbabwe and some good Zimbabwean books read during the research period.

The process of interviewing often made me rethink the aim of my stay at Sikukuchwa. Some women were in psychologically, physically and economically difficult situations. Sometimes it felt inappropriate to write down everything, when a woman just wanted to talk: an apparent tension between short and long-term objectives. My short-term objective was to provide some emotional and social support to the women. My long-term objective was the aim of the study: to understand more about the position of HIV-positive women in Zimbabwe, to assess their needs for support and to increase other's awareness. It was hard to combine these two things – reacting with empathy and listening to the women seemed at odds with writing down information and interpreting these data scientifically. What could I say to the woman who asked at the end of my interview, after answering all my questions: 'But Judith, I want to ask you a question... My husband goes around with other ladies, what can I do?' This was one of the occasions when I felt very ambivalent: thankful (because she took me into her confidence) but nonetheless powerless.

What is the relevance of this study to AIDS policy and what might it contribute to the fight against AIDS? Considering the impact of HIV infection on a specific group of women receiving a form of support may also say something about the many other women with HIV and AIDS who are and probably will remain silent, as my informants elaborated extensively on their experiences before and after they found the Sikukuchwa project. Whenever possible I have tried to place the problems that HIV-positive women at Sikukuchwa experienced within a larger social context. Further, it is my hope that insight into the consequences for women with HIV/AIDS in Zimbabwe and a deeper understanding of their individual coping responses – including the role of support – will help other organizations and persons working in the field. This Bulletin is meant to be disseminated among counsellors, policymakers and researchers who work in the area of care and support, including psychosocial areas, for women with HIV/AIDS. The description in the following chapters of the dire consequences of HIV and AIDS for women as well as the strategies they use to deal with their reality will, I hope, help those responsible for providing care and support to HIV-positive women to involve the women themselves fully in the development and implementation of activities.

The research process, from participating in daily project activities and conducting interviews up to writing an objective description of the facts back in the Netherlands, has not been easy. There are many people without whose collaboration, support and inspiration I would not have been able to finalize these tasks. First I would like to thank all of the HIV-positive women of Sikukuchwa for their frank honesty and their kind, hospitable attitude. Although they felt very downcast at times, most often they were talking and laughing. I was both amazed and thrilled by their positive attitude, and I fully admire the way they were living with illness. Some women invited me into their homes, although their families did not – and probably still do not – know the real reason for my stay in Zimbabwe. I give a special word of thanks to Tsitsi. Through our daily contact she often made me somehow understand what it really is to be HIV positive and eventually to have full-blown AIDS. I also express my sincere thanks to the coordinators at Sikukuchwa for giving me the opportunity to stay there for four months and participate in daily project activities. Their support allowed easy access to HIV-positive women; without such help this in many respects intensive research experience would not have materialized. Last but not least I thank Prof. Corlien Varkevisser for her valuable support and comments during all stages of the research, including the fieldwork, and the publication of this book. Where today can one find a professor who takes time to read, comment and discuss papers with genuine interest and allows a former student to stay and write in her garden house? Luckily, I did!

Judith van Woudenberg

Introduction

The AIDS epidemic and its consequences

We may cure AIDS, but we won't eradicate infectious disease. At best, we can keep pace, reduce suffering, and begin to examine the process by which perceptions of disease engender prejudice, social disruption, and culture change. (S.C. McCombie, AIDS in cultural, historic, and epidemiologic context, 1990)

Estimates – in which underreporting is likely – suggest that currently 8.77 million people in Sub-Saharan Africa carry the HIV virus (Mann et al., 1992). Thus while only 10% of the world's population lives in this region, more than 60% of HIV infections are found there. The percentage of HIV-infected people has reached 20–30% of the adult population in many African cities, including those of Zimbabwe. HIV/AIDS is having an enormous impact on societies, even though this is only slowly being documented.

In developing countries, the impact on women is particularly great, as will be discussed below. Improvements to their quality of life have come about mostly through their own struggles to learn how to live with HIV, from their own lived experiences (Bolton, 1992). Coping with the pandemic has been singled out by the World Health Organization/Global Programme on AIDS (WHO/GPA) as a research area deserving priority action and funding. Recommended research includes: a) documenting the psychological, social and legal consequences of HIV for individuals, families and communities, b) documenting the various ways people cope with these consequences, and c) studying the effectiveness of various experimental strategies for enhancing people's ability to cope (WHO Features, 1991).

HIV/AIDS are accompanied by psychological, social, cultural, economic and political consequences. If realistic preventive measures and effective responses to the epidemic are to be developed, better understanding of these consequences will be essential. Systematic qualitative investigation among people with HIV/AIDS can contribute substantially to the needed knowledge and understanding (Abramson and Herdt, 1990). The aim of the present publication is to share results of a medical anthropological study among women with HIV in Zimbabwe, to provide some answers to questions about how women can live with HIV and what constitutes meaningful support to those who are infected.

Social history and media presentation

When the mass media confronted the world with HIV/AIDS, sufferers were often presented as illegal and immoral (Herdt, 1992). In the West, there was a tendency to minimize the seriousness of AIDS, which was often regarded as a disease affecting those outside the mainstream of society (Barnett and Blaikie, 1992). In Africa, however, AIDS is not primarily a disease of marginalized groups. In contrast to North America and Europe where initial cases were primarily found among homosexual men, AIDS in Africa occurs in women about as often as in men. Everyone is at risk. Growing numbers of infected women mean that perinatal transmission is also of significant public health importance. Heterosexual intercourse as the major transmission mechanism in Africa appears to frighten the West; anxieties have found expression in all sorts of media explanations. People with HIV or AIDS have invariably been presented as victims, and myths, stereotypes and misplaced images of the dark continent have prevailed.

Many misunderstandings about the epidemic and those who become infected remain. To fully understand the epidemiology and consequences of AIDS in Africa we need to consider both social and biological components. The intersection among colonial history, traditional culture and present-day political economy has shaped the course of AIDS in Africa (Bassett and Mhloyi, 1991); as we see below, this includes Zimbabwe. The resulting social setting has affected both family structures and sexual relationships. Herdt (1992) rightly states that the impact of AIDS has been shaped by the social realities of Africa, and now in turn the disease is dramatically changing these realities, affecting how people live and organize their societies (Herdt, 1992).

Women and HIV/AIDS

I think my mother admired my tenacity, and also felt sorry for me because of it. She began to prepare me for disappointment long before I would have been forced to face up to it. To prepare me she began to discourage me. And do you think you are so different, so much better than the rest of us? Accept your lot and enjoy what you can of it. There is nothing else to be done. (Dangarembga, Nervous conditions, 1990, p. 20)

Women in developing countries suffer most from the epidemic. In addition to increased risk of infection and vulnerability and greater difficulty in taking preventive measures, the psychological and social conditions in which they must cope with the epidemic are potentially severe; negative portrayals and stereotypes of women in the media as well as in AIDS prevention campaigns also contribute.

Several complex socio-cultural factors make women in Africa more vulnerable to HIV. These include widow inheritance, polygamy, low power to make decisions in sexual matters, and relatively less access to adequate services and information due to relatively low levels of education (de Bruyn, 1992). Some traditional sexual practices promote unsafe sexual activities among men and increase women's risk: postpartum sexual abstinence for women, while spouses continue to have sexual contacts, put women at risk, as does the ritual cleansing ceremony after a husband's death, when the spouse is purified or frees her husband's spirit by having intercourse with a brother of the husband (de Bruyn, 1992). Socioeconomic factors which indirectly bear on women's risk include migration of husbands to urban areas to look for jobs (perhaps to return with HIV or another STD), poor nutritional status, poor hygiene, and the necessity to use sex as a economic resource (Schoepf, 1993). Moreover, girls become sexually active at a younger age than boys, and marry younger; their older partners may also be riskier. Older men specifically look for sex with younger women, hoping they are still free of HIV. Too, sexual abuse, including incest and rape, affects more girls than boys (Jackson, 1992).

Biological factors related to greater risks for women include the association between STDs and HIV and a number of factors related to pregnancy, delivery and lactation (blood transfusions, temporary immune system suppression, exposure of e.g. traditional birth attendants to HIV/AIDS). Once women have HIV, stress due to pregnancy is an additional burden; women who have lost a baby may experience increased pressure from their husband or his family to have another baby soon. HIV-positive women also risk more complications of pregnancy, and may have less access to health services than men. They may have to continue stressful household and subsistence activities even when their health is deteriorating (Jackson, 1992).

In addition to their increased risk of exposure, women's usually low socioeconomic status and lack of power relative to men (inside or outside marriage) also make it difficult for them to take preventive measures, whether HIV positive or not. Women have limited control to negotiate or enforce strategies to reduce their risk of HIV infection; they also have fewer means to prevent infection or slow down the development of AIDS. When they are in financial need, poor women who sell sexual services to supplement their income have few options if men do not wish to use condoms. Married and/or monogamous women may have steady partners who have multiple sexual contacts; though aware of this, they often are not in a position to change the situation (de Bruyn, 1992). A choice between poverty or divorce and the risk of HIV infection is a choice between 'social death' and biological death (Bassett and Mhloyi, 1991).

Inequities in the positions of men and women also make the psychological and social burdens of the disease greater for women than for men in similar situations (de Bruyn, 1992). The influence on marital and sexual relationships is particularly great. The existing age difference in sexual relationships has become more pronounced due to HIV/AIDS. Further, widows whose spouses die of AIDS may be unable to remarry, whether or not they are HIV positive. Women who have HIV or AIDS also risk rejection and divorce, with loss of social security and income as a consequence. Women also experience greater demands related to coping with the effects of the epidemic. As elsewhere, women in Africa are the main caregivers. It is their responsibility to care for the sick, which may include husbands and children infected with HIV; but there may be no one to care for them at home when they are ill. Two stereotypes are important, namely AIDS as a 'homosexual disease' and AIDS as a 'prostitute's' or 'women's' disease (de Bruyn, 1992). The effect of the first stereotype for women is particularly relevant in the West: women may not be recognized or recognize themselves as potential patients, delaying diagnosis and treatment. The second stereotype implies stigmatization, with consequences for women's socioeconomic status.

In the remainder of the Introduction these factors are examined more thoroughly in the Zimbabwean situation.

HIV and AIDS in Zimbabwe

Everybody knows that pestilences have a way of recurring in the world, yet sometimes we find it hard to believe in ones that crash down on our heads from a blue sky. There have always been as many plagues as wars in history. Yet always plagues and wars take people equally by surprise.
(Albert Camus, The plague, 1972)

HIV was first recognized in Zimbabwe in the early 1980s; the high level of other STDs in the general population was a factor in its rapid spread. Blood donor data suggested a rapid rise in infection: in 1985 on average 2.3 per cent of donors tested HIV positive; five years later, the figure in some urban areas exceeded 15 per cent (Bassett and Mhloyi, 1991). In 1991 and 1992 HIV infections among STD patients at some sites reached 60% (NACP, 1991, 1992). In some border towns, seroprevalence up to 40% has been recorded (Meursing and Sibindi, 1995). Initially, there were major reporting problems. Procedures gradually improved, but as 1990 ended reporting was still so incomplete that the Minister of Health and Child Welfare felt AIDS should be made legally notifiable (Jackson, 1992). By 1993 21,000 full-blown AIDS cases had been reported. The coordinator of the NACP (National AIDS Coordination Programme, Ministry of Health, personal communication) estimated this was only one-third of the actual number. Figure 1 shows the cumulative AIDS cases by age group and sex in the five years ending in December 1992. Two major peaks are seen, at age 20–39 (60% of AIDS cases) and among under fives (babies infected by their mothers during pregnancy or childbirth). Babies with HIV develop AIDS more quickly than adults, because their immune systems are less developed. The majority die within two or three years of birth. Further, it is striking that, as discussed above, in the younger age groups women with AIDS outnumber men, due to age differences at the onset of sexual activity.

In 1996, WHO reported Zimbabwe to be the country with the sixth highest AIDS incidence, with 41,298 reported cases (AIDS Bestrijding, 1996). This is still apt to be low with respect to the actual number, but less so than previous estimates. AIDS hits the sexually and economically active population hardest. For Zimbabwe, one of the most industrially developed countries in Africa, the epidemic has major economic implications, threatening to increase the existing shortage of skilled labour. Moreover, since most of the country's ten million people rely on the state for medical care AIDS greatly increases the burden on the public health sector (Southern Africa Economist, 1992).

Socioeconomic conditions and HIV/AIDS

The broader socioeconomic framework of Zimbabwean culture, colonial history and present-day political economy provide a context for the study presented here. As in other countries, sexual inequality is a part of this context. The consequences for women are clear; the effects on their coping with HIV/AIDS will be seen in later chapters.

Zimbabwe was colonialized nearly a century ago, a history which has

Figure 1   Cumulative AIDS cases 1987-1992 in Zimbabwe, by age and sex

Number of cases

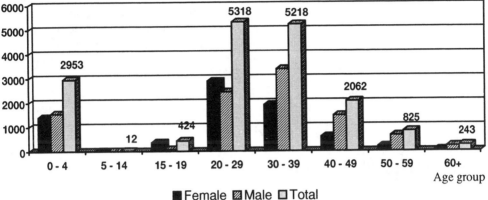

For 1505 cases, no age or sex was specified

Source: NACP, 1992

contributed to the explosive spread of HIV and other STDs. In the 1890s white pioneers entered Zimbabwe from South Africa in search of gold, but gold mining appeared unprofitable. They shifted to agriculture and began to appropriate African land. The commercial expansion of the agricultural sector and creation of a labour pool made up of landless peasants forced Zimbabweans into a cash economy. The expropriation of land continued; by the 1930s, whites comprised less than five per cent of the population but owned half of the land (Bassett and Mhloyi, 1991). The other half, Tribal Trust Lands, was allotted to indigenous people but was the least productive. As a result, women's already limited rights to ownership over the land or its products decreased still further. Since independence these areas have been called 'communal areas'; the land-less poor remain one of Zimbabwe's greatest problems.

Lack of land and rural impoverishment pushed men further into migrant labour in cities, on large-scale farms, or in mines. Wives remained in the rural home, where their farm work doubled as they took over men's activities. As marital separation became common, the instability of the family increased, leading to new patterns in sexual relations characterized by multiple partners. Initially this was limited to men, who established casual relationships near their workplaces. During their long periods of absence, the money they sent home gradually decreased. This, in addition to the loss of their labour, had a major impact on rural households. As financial resources declined, some women were forced to engage in occasional sex for money: women's migration to towns was restricted, but some, driven by poverty, migrated and began to meet the growing demand. Other women moved to town to seek formal employment or higher education. Urbanization reduced families' social control over the sexual behaviour of both men and women (Meursing and Sibindi, 1995). The multiple

11

relationships that arose in the urban setting of colonial and postcolonial Zimbabwean society differ considerably from the polygamous unions seen in traditional culture (Bassett and Mhloyi, 1991).

In 1980, Zimbabwe became independent after a long and bitter war. Today's political economy is rooted in colonial as well as traditional history. The desire to redistribute land in favour of those who had fought was expressed repeatedly after independence, but implementation has been minimal. Structural adjustment measures have led to growing discrepancies between rich and the great majority of the poor and have also affected the ability and willingness of the government to fund health and social budgets. Although the government adopted an intensive health policy on HIV/AIDS (through NACP) and extended AIDS education programmes, the needs in this area remain enormous.

Gender roles and sexual relationships

The patrilineal system of descent and inheritance in traditional Zimbabwean societies assigns a superior status to men. Early socialization by mothers, aunts and grandmothers, as well as the behaviour of male relatives, teaches women they are subordinate and must respect men's wishes. When a man wants to marry, officially his family must pay a bride price to compensate the woman's family for her labour and reproductive capacity and to show esteem.

Afterwards the wife belongs to the man's family; children become part of the male lineage. In principle, women can return to their family of origin only after divorce. Traditionally, women's property rights were extremely limited, as were rights regarding their children. They (Bassett and Mhloyi, 1991) were entitled to earnings from their own handwork, to plots where they could grow family food, and to certain gifts related to motherhood. This limited protection was further curtailed during the colonial period. Traditional patriarchal values were reinterpreted under European law, reducing women to minority status under the guardianship of fathers or husbands. Whereas laws governing the legal position of women have been adapted, it will be years before there are substantial changes in behaviour. Although in the early 1980s about half of households in rural areas were managed by women (Bassett and Mhloyi, 1991), women were rarely awarded land or rights to the products of their labour.

This intersection of traditional culture with changing social and political conditions has influenced sexual relationships and gender roles, and consequently the course of the AIDS epidemic. Gender roles and men and women's expectations and wishes related to sexual relationships are an essential part of understanding the problems these relationships present for women with HIV/AIDS, particularly in relation to preventive activities and childbearing. Relationships inside and outside marriage will be described separately, since they follow different paths; however, women can (or must) switch paths. Most Zimbabwean women marry, but many marriages do not last a lifetime. Premarital relationships may or may not lead to marriage. When one or both partners hope for marriage, there are preconditions. In the market economy of modern Zimbabwe, the bride price has a new economic meaning. Payment is substantial, and may take years to acquire (Bassett and Mhloyi, 1991). In a society with high unemployment, this is a substantial barrier for young men. For young woman, it is necessary to be fertile, modest and faithful, respectful to husband and in-laws; and healthy, to be able to work hard (Meursing and Sibindi, 1995). For women, there are expectations of no sex before marriage, though sexual relationships are unofficially tolerated. A pregnant girl, however, can expect disapproval, especially if she is still in school. In comparison, men's freedom in pre- and extramarital relationships seems unlimited, though they are supposed to take responsibility for any resulting children and for the mother.

By age 20–24, 75 per cent of women in Zimbabwe have married (Bassett and Mhloyi, 1991). While many legal barriers to women's equality were overturned by legal improvements after independence, at home men are still in charge. Gender roles are fairly rigid: a married man is the family's provider; the role of the wife is to care for the home, bear children and care for them. Her place is at home, the husband's place outside. Meursing and Sibindi (1995) note that though nowadays more and more women also have jobs outside and add to the family income, these role expectations have not changed. The commitment implicit in married life is that the man gets sexual and reproductive rights to his wife, in return providing food and shelter for her and his offspring. Decisions on family planning and number of children traditionally lie with the husband, but childbirth is an important goal of almost every marriage. Both women and men expect children when they marry: they prove a man's sexual activity and fertility, and are a woman's sexual obligation and a source of respect. Infertility causes great stress between spouses and with the husband's family: bride price is paid in the expectation of children. A marriage without children is barely viable, often ending in divorce.

For the majority of women, sexual relationships occur in the context of marriage. Traditionally, men are allowed more than one legal wife, but this is generally beyond their financial capacity. Nevertheless, the misconception that AIDS in Africa results from polygamy remains. In fact, polygamy in its original form protects against HIV rather than increasing the risk (Frank, 1992). In the reinterpreted traditional culture, men are apt to have a number of casual sexual relationships instead of a limited number of stable marriage partners. In either case, a wife cannot and does not question her husband's sexual behaviour, while she must remain faithful to the husband who through paying bride price obtained the right to her womb (Varkevisser, 1995). If a woman does question unfaithfulness, she cannot expect support or sympathy (Jackson, 1992). There are strong social sanctions for married women who engage in extramarital sex.

Non-marital relationships may be for pleasure, for affection and emotional closeness, for company and/or to secure financial support. Those who are divorced or widowed may form one or more relationships to pay for basic necessities or supplement a low income. Women are often responsible for several children, and may sell sex to meet specific obligations such as school fees. For many, sexual relationships with men – whether single sexual encounters or ongoing sexual and domestic services – are linked to economic and social survival. Bassett and Mhloyi (1991) point out that such relationships are by no means always seen as prostitution. While these patterns are widely believed to be a well established feature of towns but not rural areas, rudimentary business centres, army camps and the like also offer opportunities for exchanging sex for money or other goods and services. Younger women, even of school age, may trade sex for support from an older lovers – 'sugar daddies' – who provide otherwise inaccessible goods or experiences (meals in hotels, rides in an expensive car, and so on). Finally, employed women may be forced to exchange sex for job security (Bassett and Mhloyi, 1991). For unmarried men or those living apart from their wives, these relationships provide sex, company and perhaps someone to do the cooking and cleaning, greatly improving their quality of live without adding much responsibility. The threat of HIV has not drastically changed such sexual relationships (Meursing and Sibindi, 1995).

STDs, condoms and HIV/AIDS

As patterns of sexual networking altered, all STDs, recently including HIV, became rampant. There is a double linkage between STDs and AIDS. The presence of STDs indicates risk groups among whom HIV may be present or easily spread. In addition, STDs appear to be a cofactor in HIV transmission, so that the rapid spread of AIDS may be largely explained by high rates of STD infection. In the early 1990s, public health facilities in Zimbabwe recorded more than one million STD episodes. This means nearly one-quarter of the adult population were treated for STDs. Chancroid is of particular concern, since it accounts for about half of genital ulcer disease in Zimbabwe (Bassett and Mhloyi, 1991.

In most cases the male partner introduces HIV infection into the family unit (Bassett and Mhloyi, 1991). However, the use of condoms, in marriage or outside, depends on male willingness. Most men dislike condoms for several reasons, all related to the quality of their sexual lives. Women blame condoms for promoting promiscuity, and everyone associates them with HIV/AIDS. To prevent pregnancy, many Zimbabweans use oral contraceptives. Since the AIDS campaign began promoting (and giving free) condoms for STD/HIV prevention, distribution has greatly increased, but condoms remain highly controversial (Meursing and Sibindi, 1995).

Meursing and Sibindi (1995) found that the presence of STDs did not lead to marital crises. Discussion of STDs or condoms seldom takes place. Women often take STDs as one burden of married life, or do not dare challenge husbands, as they might lose their financial support. A woman who dares to suggest her partner should avoid risky sexual acts or use condoms often encounters male refusal, is accused of adultery or promiscuity, is suspected of already being infected with HIV, or is said to be accusing the partner of infidelity (Schoepf et al., 1988; Bledsoe, 1990). Spouses might go separately to a doctor or abstain from sex for a while. As Meursing and Sibindi (1995) note these practices are of course inadequate to prevent HIV or other STDs either before or after a positive HIV diagnosis.

AIDS education and prevention

Partly as a result of the presentation of AIDS in the worldwide media, reactions in the form of educational programmes came slowly in many African countries, including Zimbabwe. Admitting AIDS was becoming an issue seemed like admitting the inferiority of African life, and threatened the growing tourist industry (Bassett and Mhloyi, 1991). When the epidemic continued to grow the government did initiate prevention programmes, beginning a national AIDS campaign in the early 1990s. In Zimbabwe, as in many countries, the first mass national health education campaigns raised anxiety, panic and disbelief: 'Beware of AIDS, AIDS kills' and 'Make sure what you are taking home tonight is not AIDS'. These quick reactions were not carefully thought out, either by the government or by the non-governmental organizations (NGOs) who first identified the problem. The focus was on sticking to one partner and being faithful; unmarried women were perceived as potential sources of infection; and no messages were included for the many people in Zimbabwe who were already infected. People with HIV/AIDS were portrayed as victims, already dying (Ray, 1992). No singers or other artists stood up, raised awareness and promoted personal behavioural change. These campaigns were not very effective, because they did not take cultural codes and changing socioeconomic conditions into account (Meursing, 1997).

From this perspective it is not surprising that from the beginning people have been afraid of letting their HIV status be known. Stigmatization and discrimination are often aroused when people feel uncertain, have their integrity threatened or lack self confidence, as may happen in times of political uncertainty, natural disasters or health crises. The easiest way to deal with an epidemic is to put the blame elsewhere, whether on minority groups or events beyond one's control. As a consequence, AIDS becomes politicized (Farmer, 1990); taboos and secrecy result. This is exactly what happened in Zimbabwe. As a result of health education programmes and campaigns, people in Zimbabwe are now aware of HIV/AIDS. This knowledge, however, is mainly limited to ideas such as: AIDS is a problem; it cannot be cured; and one can prevent AIDS by using condoms or being faithful. As in many countries, ambivalent attitudes abound. Ignorance of risks, fatalism and prevailing sexual norms prevent people from changing their own behaviour. Further, healthy people – or, more precisely, people who do not know if they are HIV positive – tend to dissociate themselves from those suspected of being infected. It is difficult to realize that tomorrow you may belong to the very same group: perhaps due to anxiety, people cannot identify with those with AIDS, and often react with little empathy.

Dawn of a new life

In Zimbabwe, the number of people with HIV/AIDS has increased rapidly; efforts to assist have been few in comparison to their needs. Sikukuchwa Care Trust is one of the few organizations that enables HIV-positive people to do something about their own situation. Initiated (June 1990) and run by two Catholic sisters, this non-governmental organization is situated in a low-density district of

15

Harare, the capital of Zimbabwe. Sikukuchwa means 'the dawn of a new life' – a name chosen to offer inspiration to people with HIV/AIDS. In 1993, Sikukuchwa consisted of various projects chiefly for HIV-positive women, several of which are described below.

Drop-In Crisis Centre (opened June, 1990). This centre organized income-generating activities, a support group, a prayer group, a children's play group and a feeding scheme for women and their children. It also provided pre- and post-test counselling and basic medication for HIV-positive men and women. Income-generation was organized through a *cooperative*. Knitting and sewing were the main activities; women then tried to sell their products in their own communities. Other such activities included fringing carpets (which paid minimum wages) and vegetable growing. An average of 35–40 women participated in the cooperative, but their numbers were steadily increasing. A T-shirt had been designed and printed with the logo of the organization, and was being sold in various shops in and outside Harare. Women came to the centre only during the daytime, continuing to sleep at home. A *support group* (self help group) had been established in which HIV-positive women, most of whom also participated in the cooperative, could share thoughts and ideas in weekly meetings. For children under six years old of HIV-positive mothers participating in the cooperative, a pre-school teacher was employed in June 1993.

Home Based Care team (began February, 1992). The team consisted of a trained nurse, four counsellors for HIV positives who were themselves HIV-positive and a Catholic pastoral worker. They supported HIV/AIDS patients in their own homes, providing material, medical and spiritual care. Patients and family members got intensive counselling during which they were taught to care for their infected family member and for themselves. The team worked in liaison with community sisters and local clinics.

Care Unit (opened March, 1993). This four bedroom unit admitted people with full-blown AIDS. Family members or friends were the main caretakers, under the supervision of a nursing sister. When patients became terminally ill, they had to leave the unit. They could then either go back to the rural area or other place they came from, or go to a hospice of the order to which the sisters were attached, to give them a chance to die in dignity.

AIDS Awareness Programme (began June, 1990). This extensive programme provided health education talks in workplaces, schools, beer halls and churches. The educators were health care professionals, people living with HIV/AIDS, peer educators and community caregivers. HIV-positive women who participated in Sikukuchwa joined in, giving their testimony. Materials and information on AIDS were obtained from the AIDS Counselling Trust.

Orphan Outreach (started in February 1994). This programme was set up to investigate and implement a strategy for caring for children orphaned by HIV/AIDS. The aim was to avoid institutionalization by involving extended families and community members as caregivers for the children.

Since 1994, these activities have been still further extended. The study reported here was carried out within the context of the Drop-In Crisis Centre, where the Care Unit was also located. The project's overall aim was to provide assistance to women who had lost the support of their relatives and neighbours because they were HIV positive. An important objective was to re-introduce women to normal life as they shared in the income-generating activities of the cooperative and met other women in similar situations. The project aim was to keep women living in their own communities, not at Sikukuchwa, to avoid stigmatization. The project cooperated with six government clinics located in high-density areas of Harare, which referred women in need of help to the Drop-In Centre or the Home Based Care (HBC) team. Sikukuchwa also received referrals from the large hospitals in the city. The Home Based Care team in turn told HIV-positive women about the possibility of participating in the daily activities of the cooperative.

The staff of Sikukuchwa Care Trust was composed of the two Catholic sisters, both fully trained nurses and counsellors, who had initiated the project and continued to provide coordination; a Shona leader of the cooperative, who was also a local leader in the area where most women lived; and the Home Based Care team (one nurse, four counsellors for HIV positives and a pastoral worker) plus the pre-school teacher. Apart from the two sisters and the pastoral worker, who all came from Ireland, all staff members were Zimbabwean.

When visitors enter Sikukuchwa's territory, they notice that the area looks bright, open and very welcoming. Two things immediately struck me during my first week. First, the very positive atmosphere, and second, the quite central position of the two sisters coordinating the project. They were very dedicated and certainly did not stick to normal working hours. Their mandate is expressed in their mission statement.

Sikukuchwa is an independent, non-discriminatory, non-profit making orga-
nization. We are dedicated to empowering with the skills and knowledge to
deal effectively with the aids pandemic, through education and support.
Our holistic approach includes networking and a commitment to meeting
aids-related needs in the community.

1 Objectives and methodology

The intent of the study reported here was to explore the consequences of HIV infection and AIDS for HIV-positive women in Zimbabwe and the way they cope with these consequences; further, this created an opportunity to assess their need for support. Sikukuchwa Care Trust is examined here, but the conclusions and many of the observations can be extrapolated to other organizations that support people with HIV and AIDS. The potential easy access through the Sikukuchwa project was an important reason to focus on HIV-positive women. In much AIDS-related research patients drop out due to lack of time to participate in research, distance or fear that others will become aware of their problems. Daily contact with the HIV-positive women participating in the project created the trust necessary to enable me to gain insight into the issues raised by the research objectives.

Study design and constraints

Studying matters as delicate as HIV/AIDS calls for a qualitative, exploratory approach. AIDS is not only a lethal disease; it also stems from a highly stigmatized condition. What people say and do in public in relation to HIV/AIDS may differ greatly from and even contradict their private feelings and actions. For example, as will be seen later, some women who had been introduced to the project because they were positive still denied their HIV status during interviews and in other situations.

The study was conducted at Sikukuchwa in April–July 1993. The sample was composed of 19 HIV-positive women Sikukuchwa participants, who were in different stages of their disease. Data collection techniques included in-depth interviews, a focus group discussion, direct and participant observation and spontaneous, informal discussions with key informants. Because 8 of the 19 women spoke little or no English, I made use of an interpreter, who was – to maintain confidentiality – also an HIV-positive woman participant at Sikukuchwa. Data were manually processed and analysed; for a technical description, see the research report (van Woudenberg, 1994).

In reading this Bulletin it is important to realize that, in addition to the small sample size, limiting the study to women associated with the Sikukuchwa cooperative was a source of socioeconomic bias. There were no strict criteria for working in the cooperative but the women had an extremely low income and were generally unmarried or divorced. It is also possible that women at Sikukuchwa had accepted their condition to a greater degree than other women with HIV, and therefore were more stable than non-participating women in comparable positions. Because counselling and participation in a support group formed important project components, it seems likely that women in the project were accustomed to discussing their feelings relatively freely. Further, women participants were selected because they were receiving relatively little support from a partner, family and/or social environment. They were primarily recruited by the Home Based Care team, sometimes after several invitations. Eventually they dared to visit the project and meet other women in the same situation. Consequences of the lethal disease and possible support measures were likely understood more fully, as they were extensively discussed. However, not all women were socioeconomically powerless. Some whose health improved managed re-integration in society, and may then have been better off due to their Sikukuchwa experience than women who missed this opportunity.

Limitations and ethical considerations

In planning the research, a control group of HIV-positive women not participating at Sikukuchwa was intended, to give an impression of the degree to which the socioeconomic conditions of those in the project were representative and allow an assessment of the effects of the project. Due to lack of time, combined with ethical considerations, this could not be done. None of the proposed sampling techniques was possible; even women participating in the Sikukuchwa project did not reveal their HIV status, so that it would have been very difficult for them to identify (or for me to approach) HIV-positive women who were not receiving support from Sikukuchwa. Further, confidentiality made it totally impossible to use records from the hospitals used by the HIV-positive women at Sikukuchwa to set up a control group. Due to the limited registration of HIV-positive people, it was also not possible to compare the demographic characteristics of HIV-positive women in the general population to those of the sample. The NACP records only the number of cumulative AIDS cases by age and sex. As Figure 1 in the Introduction makes evident, AIDS is especially prevalent among women aged 20–29. The sample does correspond with this finding, as the mean age was 27.8 years and most women (12) were aged 20–29.

Another source of concern is related to difficulties in summarizing and interpreting responses. As every woman had her own story, life events and unique response to AIDS it proved difficult to make general statements even for this small sample. However, in many respects the HIV-positive women at Sikukuchwa found themselves in comparable positions. The degree of consensus in the group was also remarkable. Women often had similar opinions and seemed to act similarly. This may in part originate in the intensive exchange of information and experiences and the strong emotional bond among the women, and in turn these group dynamics may have prevented assessing the individual opinions on HIV/AIDS of some less outspoken women. Further, although I have tried to describe the process of coping with HIV/AIDS over a span of time, three months of field research is not long enough to cover all consequences. Most women had experienced a long history of sickness and would face new problems in the future. Many women were especially willing to share their experiences with me when experiencing problems. The interviews and observations reflect what was going on in their lives at particular moments.

In addition to limitations in the data, the still greater problem lies in the translation of experiences or emotions into words. The words of Tsitsi, a woman with full-blown AIDS, illustrate this: 'They'll never understand – even you.' The limitations of behavioural research become particularly clear in studying a subject such as HIV/AIDS. The most emotional, complex and intimate feelings dealing with sexual or other relationships and death must be translated into rational words on a piece of paper. Also, some feelings have no adequate equivalent in the Shona language; as a consequence, women had to describe instead of simply stating their feelings. Moreover, Zimbabweans generally do not talk about feelings as much as in many Western societies. On the other hand, while in Western societies people often rationalize feelings while being unwilling to show them, the reverse seems true in Shona culture. In any case, to me a human being seems to a large extent a product of thoughts, ideas, values, norms, experiences, expectations and emotions so complex they can hardly be described. Therefore, this Bulletin can provide only an approximation to the condition in which HIV-positive women participating in the Sikukuchwa project found themselves. The reader should see it as a rather rational (thus simplified) description of the complex reality of women living with HIV or AIDS. Each woman's story is unique.

Theoretical background

Attitudes and behaviour in relation to HIV/AIDS

Numerous studies of knowledge, attitudes and behaviour (KABP studies) concerning HIV/AIDS have been conducted in various countries. Insight in these areas can help predict the degree of tolerance and acceptance persons with HIV/AIDS are apt to experience, as well as the ways people will protect themselves (or not) against infection. Pitts et al. (1990) provide particularly interesting results of interviews with social workers. Generally speaking, this group appears to display high levels of knowledge and positive attitudes towards people with HIV/AIDS. However, detailed examination of responses showed gaps in knowledge, plus ambivalent attitudes and behaviours. Adamchak et al. (1990) indicated reasonably high knowledge of AIDS among currently married Zimbabwean men, although behavioural change to avoid contracting AIDS appeared relatively low. A finding that knowledge does not necessary relate to behaviour is common (Laver, 1993; van Woerkom, 1987; Kok, 1987).

Myths, stereotypes and discrimination

Given the distorted picture of HIV/AIDS in the media and among some scientists as well, public myths and stereotypes about causes are not surprising. The wasting syndrome 'slim disease' was described in Uganda in the early 1980s (Bassett and Mhloyi, 1991); as a result people decided whether they could trust their partner or not based on outward appearance. Schoepf et al. (1988) reported that in Zaire people initially joked about AIDS as an 'imaginary syndrome invented by Europeans to discourage African lovers'. And in Zimbabwe, 'AIDS was created by the Western media to stigmatize Africa again' and 'AIDS is a threat created by churches to frighten us against loose sex' (Jackson, 1992). In Zimbabwe, some popular ideas about STDs conflict with health education messages, since they suggest that for a man, having an STD is a proof of sexual activity and manhood (Bassett and Mhloyi, 1991).

Among the factors affecting women are traditional ideas about diseases associated with AIDS, pinpointing women as transmission vectors (de Bruyn, 1992): STDs as 'women's diseases'; ideas that women who have been aborted or miscarried but not 'cleansed' can pollute men or transmit AIDS by witchcraft (Bledsoe, 1990); or of AIDS as linked to other diseases that can be caused by malign magic (Farmer, 1990). As noted in the Introduction, stereotypes – particularly of AIDS as a prostitutes' disease – also have negative consequences for women. This has an epidemiological basis, but is wrongly interpreted to mean that without female sex workers there would be no AIDS epidemic (Bassett and Mhloyi, 1991); the role of infectious male clients is still ignored. Such 'blaming' is reinforced by stigmatizing depictions (as sinful and deviant) that have found their way into AIDS control programmes. An early poster in Zimbabwe depicted a woman in a miniskirt and high-heeled boots, dragging on a cigarette; the caption exhorted men to remain faithful to their families (Bassett and Mhloyi, 1991). Their low social position, combined with presentations in the media, often singles out African women. A highly unfortunate consequence is that urban women in general, particularly if divorced or unmarried, are seen as almost synonymous with prostitutes, and thus potentially infectious. Some women who only occasionally engage in sex as a source of income will avoid condom use to avoid being identified as prostitutes. Another consequence is that women may avoid HIV testing, decreasing the chance of appropriate treatment for opportunistic infections and increasing their risk of early mortality if they are seropositive (de Bruyn, 1992).

Psychosocial consequences

Psychological consequences of HIV and AIDS have been less explored than other facets. Jackson (1991) pointed out that a diagnosis of HIV or AIDS may mean very different things for different families or individuals. AIDS can affect whole families; no one is prepared for the death of one or more children, followed by the death of both parents – let alone death caused by a highly stigmatized condition. People fired by employers due to HIV/AIDS can be robbed of dignity, selfrespect and purpose in life (Jackson, 1991). Sibanda (1990) reported respondents' feelings of uncertainty, loss of internal control, frustration and anxiety related to HIV. Berer and Ray (1993) noted that uncertainty may be the most difficult aspect of infection or disease to cope with. Fear, stress, depression, isolation and feeling unable to manage a situation affect everyone, especially people who are ill, feel they have no control or may become ill at any time. Women may be particularly susceptible to stress and depression, or at least seek help for these more often than men. Fear of rejection often leaves women afraid to tell anyone or seek help. As a result, many feel isolated and alone. Worldwide, anxieties of people with HIV/AIDS observed by Berer and Ray include risk of infecting others; social and sexual hostility and rejection; abandonment; inability to change their circumstances; insecurity about ensuring the best possible future physical health; the possibility of repeated or new infections; the inability of their environment to cope with their problems; insecurity about availability of appropriate medical treatment; possible loss of privacy and confidentiality; and loss of physical and financial independence.

Socioeconomic consequences

Research on socioeconomic consequences for individuals is almost exclusively limited to the detailed study of Barnett and Blaikie (1992). These authors stress that AIDS affects the age group which is not only sexually but also economically most active. In general, the producer/consumer ratio in *afflicted* and *affected* households[1] changes unfavourably. There are direct consequences for households due to medical expenses and loss of income as patients and those caring for them become less productive or lose jobs. This drains family resources, resulting in a lower standard of living, less nutritious food, and decreases in life expectancy. Children may have to leave school because fees cannot be paid and their labour is needed. AIDS robs children of their parents, elderly are deprived their children's care and of a decent burial, families face extinction as young people die childless, and fear of infection strains relationships (Barnett and Blaikie, 1992). How households survive depends on their resources – labour, land, cash reserves, income-generating activities and skills (including caring and managing the household). Social resources, mainly networks of material and emotional support (including the number of close relatives left and how much they can help), may become more important. As Barnett and Blaikie (1992) point out, the position of the household in the demographic cycle as well as its socioeconomic position influence access to these resources.

The generally low socioeconomic position of women accords HIV/AIDS a profound economic impact. Women with AIDS are often abandoned by their husbands, even if he was the source of infection (Kaleeba, 1989). In many African societies women do not have the same legal rights as men – a divorced woman may be left without any means of support (Willmore, 1990). Widows have similar problems. When a husband dies of AIDS, she may be unable to remarry, whether she is HIV positive or not; she faces an uncertain, impoverished future (de Bruyn, 1992). Having no diplomas, most women are virtually excluded from formal sector employment. As Barnett and Blaikie (1992) have noted, women therefore are often self-employed, producing crafts, vending food or beer, or sex work. They observe that the majority of widows stay in their marital homes, supporting themselves and their dependants. Others migrate to town, re-marry or return to their parents. Many older widows turn to celibacy and religion. Most remain impoverished, struggling for the day-to-day survival of themselves and their children (Schoepf, 1992).

Coping with a life event

Although substantial research has been carried out on coping behaviour in general, relatively little information is available about coping with HIV/AIDS. The term 'coping' has been used in various ways; in this Bulletin it is a general term including defence mechanisms, active ways of solving problems and methods for handling stress (Murphy and Moriarty, 1976). Barnett and Blaikie (1992) clearly explain the process: coping deals with the ways we all change when we realize that 'normality' has changed into 'abnormality', so that our normal expectations of life must be adjusted. Recognizing that such a transition has occurred, we seek explanations and courses of action that will enable us to achieve solutions we find culturally and personally significant. These processes require us to develop practical strategies for coping, as well as language and concepts to manage the new situation.

In the early step of coping with a disease or crisis by 'explaining' it, most people use a combination of rational responses with others that may be seen as non-rational (Barnett and Blaikie, 1992). These may in fact be based on different rationales (chance, luck, witchcraft, sorcery, sin, punishment for moral misdemeanour); they are thus not *ir*rational. One culture may reject a response as irrelevant, while to another it is plausible, logical behaviour. Traditional values and cultural concepts related to dealing with disease always play a role in coping with HIV and AIDS, and people's subjective understanding of their own illness always goes beyond physical or biomedical explanations. Schüssler (1992) uses the term *illness concept*, understood to comprise culturally accepted interpretations, explanations and predictions with regard to one's health status. How significant an illness becomes for an individual reflects one's personal experience, knowledge and cultural inheritance. One's pre-existing framework provides codes and norms for dealing with disease, including for example those related to having sex given the threat of STDs. For example, in Uganda men tend to close their eyes to risky behaviour; women more often see AIDS as a threat to themselves and their children, against which there is little defence given their subjection to men (Varkevisser, 1993). Rules for communicating and talking about diseases may thus greatly influence the impact of preventive measures. They may also determine whether direct support is available. In many African countries the custom is to inform your family when you have a serious disease (Meursing, personal communication). HIV, however, creates ambiguities: the virus is deadly, but one can live with it for many years. People have different ways to deal with HIV/AIDS; these influence general discussions as well as decisions about revealing HIV status.

Barnett and Blaikie (1992) distinguish two prerequisites for coping: 1) before a crisis can be coped with, it must be recognized and identified in a way that means something to the people affected; and 2) there needs to be a stable basis for decisions based on a social, economic and natural environment that is not too turbulent. However, the AIDS pandemic is unprecedented. AIDS is a gradual disaster, not a discrete event with known stages and subsequent responses like earthquakes or droughts. Confronted by uncertainty and seeking to normalize the situation, people will undertake a range of 'experiments' as their experience increases. Farmer describes this process in rural Haiti from the beginning of the epidemic until six years later. Local understanding of AIDS as interpreted in old conceptual frameworks was replaced by an entirely new cultural model: a new disease that might affect anyone. According to Barnett and Blaikie, AIDS as a long term disaster extends and delays coping stages. Normal coping mechanisms do not immediately show signs of stress; only with an unprecedented number of deaths do existing mechanisms begin to seem inadequate. These conclusions reinforce those of Farmer, who states that the mobilization of new coping responses takes at least five years. By the time AIDS syndromes are recognized, infection is widespread; people are suffering and dying. Care of the sick, support for orphans and other relatives, funerals and so forth clearly cannot follow established patterns. Yet prior planning is impossible; adaptations must be based on experience.

Essential needs of women living with HIV and AIDS

- encouragement, support and funding to establish and develop self-help groups and local and international networks of women living with HIV/AIDS;
- realistic media portrayals, instead of stigmatizing ones;
- equitable, accessible and affordable treatment and research regarding the effect of HIV on women (including psychosocial and medical aspects, and both complementary and allopathic treatments);
- funding for services and support for women living with HIV/AIDS, to alleviate their isolation and meet their basic needs (with evaluation and monitoring to ensure that women actually benefit);
- the right to make their own choices about reproduction and be respected and supported in those choices (including the right to have children or not);
- recognition of the right of their children and orphans to care, and of the importance of their role as parents;
- education and training of health care providers and the community at large about women's risks and needs (up-to-date, accurate information on all issues of women living with HIV/AIDS should be readily available);
- recognition of the fundamental human rights of all women living with HIV/AIDS, with special consideration for women in prison, drug users and sex workers;
- research into woman to woman transmission, and recognition of and support for lesbians living with HIV/AIDS;
- decision making power, with consultation at all levels of policy and programmes affecting women living with HIV/AIDS;
- economic support for women living with HIV/AIDS in developing countries, to help them to be self-sufficient and independent;
- inclusion of clinical manifestations specific to women in any definition of AIDS.

Source: ICWLA, 1992

Psychosocial consequences of HIV infection and the ways patients and families cope was the subject of a study in Bulawayo, Zimbabwe, which suggested that (while informing sexual partners and relevant family or community members could be an important step in coping with HIV) almost half of patients with steady partners did not inform them. Fear of rejection and loss of support were the most common reasons (Meursing and Sibindi, 1993). In 1995, Meursing and Sibindi showed few Zimbabwean couples ever mentioning HIV to each other as something that might happen to them, until they were diagnosed as HIV positive. Sibanda (1990) found earlier that affiliation with a philanthropic organization had a positive effect on coping abilities. Knowing someone else who is HIV positive seemed to enhance coping, as more than one-third who had had contact with others with HIV reported being better able to cope.

Needs for support

Since little information on consequences of and coping with HIV/AIDS was available when I conducted my study, there was scant research-based knowledge about needs among people with HIV/AIDS or the manner in which support could be provided, in particular for women. Yet people are likely to need information, understanding and social support, including that for emotional problems related

24

to accepting a diagnosis. On a practical level, they have material and financial needs as well as increasing needs for medical and nursing care as physical health declines. The range of needs must be individually assessed (Jackson, 1991). Sibanda (1990) reported the majority of people with AIDS saying their immediate needs were someone to talk to and information concerning the syndrome. Meursing and Sibindi's (1993) findings showed a variety of needs among people with AIDS or HIV, including interventions in conflicts and social support, assistance in legal and work-related issues, and emotional support. As a result of clients' tendencies to hide problems or look for help without revealing their HIV status, some sources of help are actually under-utilised (Meursing and Sibindi, 1993).

Women need greater access to information about HIV/AIDS plus support networks. At a pre-conference before the eighth International AIDS Conference (1992), seropositive women from 30 countries established a network – the International Community of Women Living with HIV/AIDS (ICWLA). Their view of the needs of women living with HIV and AIDS is summarized under 'Essential needs...' on page 24. After this conference, many initiatives were designed to address these needs (Berer and Ray, 1993; KIT, SAfAIDS and WHO joint report, 1995).

Interventions for people with HIV/AIDS and relatives

When the work described in this Bulletin was underway, most studies intended to facilitate the development of an AIDS intervention project had the objective of gathering basic information about knowledge, attitudes and practices in relation to AIDS. As a result, most interventions were directed towards AIDS awareness, education and prevention campaigns. Before 1992, research on support for interventions intended especially for HIV-infected women and their families covered diverse issues such as medical aid (Chibatamoto et al., 1992; Dehne, 1989), needs of orphans (UNICEF, 1991; Chinemana, 1992), home based care (Jackson, 1992; Manyame, 1991; CADEC, 1991), and community based self-help and support groups for women (Chinemana, 1992). After 1992, as mentioned earlier, many interventions were directed at women living with HIV/AIDS (Berer and Ray, 1993; KIT, SAfAIDS and WHO joint report, 1995).

Jackson (1992) found the majority of HIV/AIDS patients seen at a hospital in Zimbabwe were sent back home, on the assumption that somehow they would be able to look after themselves. However, some patients need support: home based care can be a solution. When the ideals of home care are realized, such care can include medical and nursing care, training for caregivers, counselling and psychosocial support, spiritual or pastoral support, material, financial and practical support, and referral to relevant organizations (Jackson, 1992). This holistic concept suggests support for the entire family. Home care also has a preventive aspect: family and community members learn about AIDS and how to avoid it. Overall, by the end of 1992, over 40 home based care programmes reaching AIDS patients were operational in at least 22 districts and 14 urban centres of Zimbabwe. However, the ideals require substantial resources – transport, materials and staffing (Jackson, 1992). Not all projects provide all support included in the home care model.

Help need not all come from outside: HIV-infected persons and close relatives can also organize themselves to support each other. Self-help groups are usually formed by peers who come together for mutual assistance in a common need, to overcome a common handicap or life-disrupting problem and bring about desired social and personal change (Katz and Bender, 1976). Self-help groups offer compensatory social ties, counteracting feelings of loneliness and uniqueness by creating a sense of community (Gottlieb, 1988). Self-disclosure is a predominant form of communication in self-help groups (Stewart, 1990): the findings of Pennebaker et al. (1988) suggest the disclosure of traumas is associated with improvement in certain aspects of immune function and physical health. There is growing support for the view that psychosocial stress can have immunosuppressive effects (Darko, 1986). By supplementing or substituting for deficient natural networks, self-help groups may have an immunocompetence-maintaining capacity (Stewart, 1990).

Many self-help groups of HIV-positive women have been formed (Berer and Ray, 1993); their numbers are still increasing. At the time of my study, research in Zimbabwe aimed at exploring the potential for community-based self-help and support groups for women was ongoing. For example, Chinemana (1992) worked with groups and communities of women to develop strategies, techniques and alternative mechanisms through which women could inform themselves and other girls and women about HIV and AIDS. In addition to the personal benefits, self-help groups are beneficial in supporting socioeconomic coping. Grandparents, aunts and uncles will increasingly have to shoulder the burden of AIDS orphans; how long they will be able to cope remains to be seen. New support must be provided within communities, as institutions cannot hope to cope when the extended family network fails to do so (Jackson, 1991; Barnett and Blaikie, 1992). This means that self-help groups' tendency to support self-disclosure is essential – without this communities will not know about the needs of people with HIV or AIDS or their families, and thus will have no opportunity to react.

2 Changes in personal conditions due to HIV/AIDS

If a snake comes into your house do not waste time asking where the snake came from, but kill it first and ask questions afterwards. (Ugandan saying cited by Noerine Kaleeba, We miss you all, 1991)

Knowledge of and attitudes towards HIV/AIDS (as well as the perceived cause of the HIV infection) can influence coping ability, as well as the ways people seek treatment and social or other support. This chapter describes the socioeconomic backgrounds of HIV-positive women in the Sikukuchwa project and their perceptions of HIV and AIDS (illness concepts). The last two sections address women's treatment-seeking behaviour and medical history, including counselling and referral to Sikukuchwa. This makes it possible to understand more of the women's medical background and the implications of HIV and AIDS for them. Quotations from interviewees illustrate the following chapters. In each section, especially relevant information follows each woman's name the first time it appears. These characteristics are summed up in Annex 1, with an index that makes it possible to follow an individual through the chapters.

The project

The Sikukuchwa project has many visitors. At first, some are a bit scared: they do not know what to expect of the atmosphere and the people. But – primarily because of the positive attitude of the women themselves – one day is enough to make visitors feel at ease with a stigmatized, deadly disease. From Monday to Thursday women come to Sikukuchwa, where one can see them talking and making jokes, drinking tea, eating sadza, playing with the children and working very hard. At first glance, nothing seems wrong. Yet they all have a frightening disease that cannot be cured. This reality can only be seen during a prolonged stay, with disturbances in daily activities – perhaps a woman is ill or a baby dies. Talking with women individually, it becomes clear that the optimistic faces hide a great deal of distress.

Socioeconomic background of women participants

Age. The sample of women, all with HIV or AIDS, consisted of 19 women; their mean age was 27.8 years, with a range from 19 to 42 years. Two-thirds were aged 20–29.

Ethnic group. Fourteen women belonged to various Shona groups (7 Czezuru, 4 Manyika; the rest were Mabudya, Korekore or Karanga); one woman was from the Ndebele tribe. The other four originally came from Malawi and Mozambique, though three had lived in Harare for a long time, two since they were born.

Table 1   **Income sources of interviewees**

Cate-gory	Main source of income	Number of women		Additional income sources	Economic support from relatives
		Per source	Total		
1	Welfare organizations		5	2 (1 vegetable sales/1	
	- Government Social Welfare	4		vegetable sales + knitting)	
	- Church	1			
2	Sikukuchwa		3		partial
3	Relatives		5	2 (1 sewing/1 Welfare + church)	5
4	Own income		3	1 (sewing)	
	- AIDS Awareness Programme	2			
	- Home Based Care	1			1
5	Husband's income	3		1 (Welfare + church + own income)	2
	TOTAL	19		6	9

Place of residence. Most women (13) lived in high-density suburbs around Harare. For various reasons, four more or less lived at Sikukuchwa; two others lived in the same area. Twelve lived with one or more relatives, either a husband, husband and his parents, husband's parents (the husband having died), their own parents or an older brother. Seven were still living on their own (including the four at Sikukuchwa).

Place and family of origin. Most women originally came from outside Harare, but had been in the city for some time – on average 9.9 years. Roughly half had been born and raised in a rural area, coming to Harare after marriage for work (either their own or the husband's), or recently, for medical treatment. Of seven born and raised in Harare, most had moved temporarily to other places for education, marriage or work. Two came from Mutare and Rusape, two smaller towns in Zimbabwe. Most were from big families: fifteen with five or more children, although two women had no brothers or sisters. Most families (14) were no longer complete, due to separation of parents (5) or death of one or more close relatives. Although life expectancy is quite high (about 61 years) in Zimbabwe, nine women had already experienced the death of a mother, father, sister or brother (Bossema, 1990). One woman had lost four brothers and sisters (two due to AIDS) and another two (both due to AIDS). For one nineteen year old, both parents had passed away; since then she had lived with her elder brother. The mother of another woman had died when she was five, and she had no contact with her father (he had not been married to her mother).

Education. The average educational level of the women was quite high in comparison to national averages. Eight had had four to seven years of primary education. Ten had followed secondary education, of whom five completed O-levels. Only one was illiterate. Six spoke no English. Most had ceased education because there was no money (9) or when they became pregnant (3).

Religion. Women who were religious were all Christian (18). Most were Roman Catholic (11); seven attended one of the new independent churches (Apostolic Faith Church, Forward in Faith, Zion Christian Church, the Zimbabwean Symbols of God or the Church of Zambia) and one woman said she was not religious. These new churches emphasize inspiration and relevation from the Holy Spirit. Prophecy under the inspiration of the Holy Spirit and faith healing are central features. Historically, these churches are related to what in South Africa is called the Zionist movement. Their names usually refer to Zion or the Apostles, to establish an association with the founders of Christianity (Bourdillon, 1987).

Marital status. Five women were married at the time of the interview. Five had been divorced (three due to HIV), three were widowed (their husband died of AIDS) and six were single. Four had boyfriends; of these one was divorced, one widowed and the other two single.

Children. Most women (14) had children – on average 2.6. Only two had never had children. Eight had lost children, most due to AIDS; three of these were childless as a result.

Past occupation and income. Most women (16) had no formal occupation before coming to Sikukuchwa. Most (13) had been married and said they had been just sitting at home, taking care of the kids. One had done voluntary work. Of the 9 who had had some personal income, 8 sold vegetables. One had also sewed and knitted at home. Two had also sold sexual services when single. One had worked in homes and shops, but not formally, and had also sold sex. Only three women had a more formal occupation before coming to Sikukuchwa. They worked respectively as a housegirl, a storekeeper and an employee of a tobacco farm; the last had also sold sex.

Economic condition. At Sikukuchwa, all HIV-positive women (except those with AIDS) acquired some income through the cooperative. However, this was certainly not enough to live on; most women had additional income sources and/or economic support from relatives. Table 1 categorizes women's sources of income when interviewed. All other categories were relatively better off than groups 1 and 2, whose standard of living was very low. By group:

1. Five women had absolutely minimum living standards. All lived on their own (3 divorced, 2 single), with most income from government Social Welfare or the church. There was no relative who contributed. Two sold vegetables for extra income to pay rent on their living space. Because they could not manage otherwise, two women lived at Sikukuchwa.

2. Of the three women who were completely dependent on Sikukuchwa, one had full-blown AIDS and lived in the Care Unit. Although her mother cared for her, she was economically dependent on support from Sikukuchwa. Two others lived on the income earned through the Sikukuchwa cooperative alone, without support from relatives. One of these lived with her husband, who could no longer work. The other was single and lived with parents, but the relationship was not good and they did not support her.

3. Five women relied largely on relatives for housing, food and money: one lived with her husband and his parents, two with parents and one with an older brother who was working. One woman living with her parents tried to earn by sewing at home, independent of Sikukuchwa. The fifth lived with her husband's parents; she received some support from them, plus Social Welfare and the church.

4. Three women had income sources that were independent, though linked to Sikukuchwa. Two testified in AIDS Awareness Programmes; one was a counsellor for Sikukuchwa's Home Based Care team. The latter also earned some money sewing at home. All but one also received money from relatives. The one who did not get support lived at Sikukuchwa, mainly because her mother lived too far away.

5. Three women's income came mainly from husbands. Two had husbands with a formal occupation (industrial labour), who provided a modest income for wife and children. They were to some extent able to satisfy their own needs and were less dependent on Sikukuchwa, welfare or relatives. One woman received a little income from each of three categories – her husband, her own income (testifying in AIDS Awareness Programmes) and the church plus Social Welfare.

Illness concepts

The concept of 'illness' refers to interpretations, explanations and predictions with regard to one's health status (Schüssler, 1992). Every woman has a subjective understanding of her own illness. The meaning HIV/AIDS assumes reflects her personal experience and knowledge, and the perceived cause of infection, knowledge and attitude towards HIV/AIDS influence the manner of coping and course of the disease.

Perceived cause of HIV infection

Women's perception of the cause of HIV infection is related to the way they cope: in general, the explanatory model they use for their illness can be either internally or externally oriented. The degree to which women see themselves as having some control is relevant: feelings of control or lack of it also affect the ways they cope with the disease, as does the degree to which they feel responsible. Though most women interviewed had had limited options regarding control over their own risk of infection, they perceived the cause quite neutrally, often saying they saw HIV as a responsibility shared with their husbands. A woman who was tested and found to HIV positive first, before her partner, was often blamed by him for being the source of infection. Although I did not ask the cause of infection directly (since this could have a stigmatizing effect and arose feelings of blame), eleven women mentioned it themselves. All presented a rational, biomedical explanation, saying they had been infected via sexual intercourse. Other explanatory models and non-rational responses such as bad luck, punishment or sorcery were not given in any direct way; in bad times, though, such alternative illness concepts became more significant, as will be seen in the section on treatment-seeking behaviour. Most women who were open about how they acquired the infection thought it was through a husband or boyfriend. Sometimes they blamed their spouses or other women:

I got married to this man who gave me the virus. (Nyasha, 26, widowed/boyfriend)

Men go out and with other women they can get diseases. (Tessa, 23, married)

Because I was a virgin before I met the white man, I know I got it from him. (Ann, 23, single)

My husband gave the fault to me and the quarrel went on. I said: how can I be the one, when you had the STD first? So later he thought of that and agreed. (Auxillia, 39, married)

Remarkably, most were quite neutral about the cause and viewed it, like Sarah, as a problem of both men and women. Only few saw themselves as responsible.

My husband is worried now, saying he brought it to me. (Sarah, 23, married)

I had a bad life in Mbare, I was a bad girl. I also lived with a man who was drunk all the time and he stole my money. I had many boyfriends for the money. We call it prostitution and probably I got the virus from them. (Noerine, 31, single)

Noerine indirectly took responsibility for her infection. In Chapter 5, *Long term coping strategies*, we see that this could enhance her coping ability, because it gives a feeling of internal control. Taking too much responsibility, however, could have a paralysing effect, due to feelings of shame or guilt. Of the other three former sex workers, one did not want to say anything about the cause, while the other two thought it came from their husbands:

I think from my husband, because he worked out too much. He was not used to stay in one place (where he had girlfriends). But his parents said I brought the disease to their son (Tsitsi, 31, widowed)

I think my husband had the virus and knew it. He ran away when I was one month pregnant. He has got another wife, so he went back to her. When our daughter died he didn't come. (Tendai, 42, divorced)

Knowledge about HIV and AIDS

When their blood sample was taken, most did not know much about HIV/AIDS. After coming to Sikukuchwa their knowledge improved considerably; some indicated this was very important. It helped them to feel strong, be self-confident and feel relaxed: knowledge tended to enhance feelings of control over the illness.

The day the doctor told me my child was HIV positive, I didn't know what it meant. (Tendai)

Because of knowledge I'm here at Sikukuchwa with a relaxed mind. At that time I knew nothing about HIV and AIDS, but the doctor gave me some pamphlets to read. (Nyasha)

But if you're tested and counselled, you know how it can get to you. (Tessa)

Knowledge about HIV and AIDS was quite high among the women. All knew, like Barbara, that HIV is mainly sexually transmitted, that you must use condoms both to prevent transmission to others and to protect yourself, and, as she also explained, most were also able to indicate how HIV is not transmitted; sometimes this knowledge was very specific.

You must use condoms to protect yourself. For the virus that my husband had got could get inside my blood and become bigger and bigger, so you will get more sick... If you're just living together [i.e. not having sex], you can't give the disease to others. (Barbara)

I know these days about AIDS that it's a disease caused by sexual intercourse and by blood transfusion. And also that it's a new disease, but when people are diagnosed, it doesn't mean that's the end of the life. You need to change your lifestyle, and also sexual behaviour. Control yourself. Also it needs healthy food to eat and also not to think too much. And also it needs support, you need to gather with some others and share problems, how you can stay being positive. This is a new disease, what I know about it, it's increasing. The number of people who are diagnosed is becoming higher and higher. (Ann)

If you're HIV positive there's a certain part of your body which can suffer for a long time, without any rest: eyes, stomach, leg, any part of the body. (Helen)

The women also knew some things to do to stay healthy, mostly related to food and drink. Some women took a few preventative measures to protect family and others:

I want to eat oranges and apples. (Marita)

I was drinking beer, but now I know that drinking beer is dangerous for HIV. (Tendai)

I cut my nails with a razor-blade, no one else is going to use it and I keep it away from them. If I bathe, I wipe the bath, when I have cuts. (Tessa)

When I have a wound, I always try to dab it myself. (Judy)

When I asked what they knew about the prognosis for their disease a few said they did not want to think about it. As a result they gave short answers and did not want to know more about AIDS:

I know AIDS is there. (Thandi)

At present I know nothing. That's because I'm fit and strong. (Barbara)

I don't want to think of the future. The problem I got for my child [who contracted AIDS], *I don't forget. (Sarah)*

On the other hand, five women emphasized the possibility of a long life with HIV – knowledge that might influence their coping ability.

You can live many years without getting sick. If you stay healthy, it will take maybe tomorrow, maybe five years. I live with that you don't know. (Judy)

It cannot be cured, everybody's dying, if it's your time. If the time of death has not arrived, you can live for many years. Others who are not affected can also die any moment. (Tessa)

Attitudes towards HIV infection and the disease AIDS

In this respect our townsfolk were like everybody else, wrapped up in themselves. In other words they were humanists: they disbelieved in pestilences. A pestilence isn't a thing made to man's measure: therefore we tell ourselves that pestilence is mere bogey of the mind, a bad dream that will pass away. (Albert Camus, The plague, 1972)

The first interview always started with the question 'Why are you here?' For me this was a way of finding out if a woman knew and had accepted her HIV status or not. Most immediately said they (12) or their child (5) were HIV positive. Those with an affected child knew they too were positive, having been tested after the child's diagnosis. Although there seemed to be a high degree of acceptance, two denied their HIV status during interviews, indicating they were not sure of their status. Helen said the doctor told her she should go to Sikukuchwa, without giving her results:

What happened was that she told me that she'd take me the blood, but she didn't give me the results. The problem which sent me here is that my father and mother also died. The doctor wanted to help me. (Helen, 19, boyfriend)

This may have been a way of coping, e.g. *denial* (discussed in Chapter 5, *Long term coping strategies*). To find out her HIV status, she could have asked the hospital or could have asked Sikukuchwa for another test, but she took neither initiative. 'Not knowing' left her room for doubt. This led to various statements during interviews:

I'm fit and strong. I think I'm all right.. (11 May 1993)
Now I'm thinking: if I'm HIV positive, it's okay, if I'm not, it's okay. (11 May 1993, later in the same interview)
Yes, I think I'm HIV positive, but I'm not sure. If I'm not taken by any doctor, I don't feel I'm HIV positive. So I want to see another doctor to make sure I'm HIV positive. (28 June 1993)
Me, I think I'm all right. (28 June 1993, later in the same interview)

From the moment she came to Sikukuchwa she alternated between acceptance and denial. Three months later she seemed to accept her condition to some extent. Pretty, however, was completely in denial, yet she wanted me to interview her. When she asked 'when will you interview me', Nyasha gave her opinion. Pretty did not pay much attention and we did the interview. Her answer to 'Why are you here', is given below, as is her response when I once asked if she actually knew her status. Helen and Pretty's comments caused me to drastically adapt their interviews, since most questions were directed to HIV-positive women who knew and accepted their condition. I could not assess whether either really perceived herself as HIV negative.

Judith only interviews HIV-positive women. (Nyasha, 26, widowed/boyfriend)

I was just sitting at home doing nothing. So Amai K. [leader of the cooperative] asked me to come. At the cooperative they needed someone who can learn to knit. Someone who is negative to continue the project. (Pretty, 21, divorced/ boyfriend)

I'm both sides, because we're the same. Because it's today's life, everybody's facing HIV. I think three quarters of Zimbabwe is HIV positive. (Pretty)

People with HIV or AIDS cannot hope for rapid change in their suffering, especially not if they live in a developing country. The lack of affordable treatment options influences individual's perception of their disease situation (Schüssler, 1992) and the way they deal with their illness. Women at Sikukuchwa were encouraged to adopt an illness concept of HIV in which they were not victims and could do something about their situation. Perhaps surprisingly, most women realized there was, at the time, no cure for AIDS. Even now, with some possibilities beginning to appear, the cost is still prohibitive. Appropriate counselling, medical treatment for opportunistic infections and social support remain the only feasible means to support the majority of people with HIV/AIDS. Three women however said they sometimes hoped for a cure and a prolongation of life; for example:

Judith, are you sure there isn't a medicine against AIDS in Holland? (Tsitsi, 31, widowed) (who developed full-blown AIDS during my stay)

Maybe the medicine will be found, when I'm still alive and I will be better, be cured. (Chipo, 26, married)

Medical history

Testing and counselling

Most women learned they were HIV positive because they or their baby became ill and the doctor advised a blood test. Tests took place in a hospital (14) or at Sikukuchwa (3, two after referral from a clinic); two women did not talk about their tests. The mean period since first knowledge of HIV status was 14 months; the range was three months to three years. Zimbabwean policy is for the doctor to give HIV test results to the patient, with information about the disease and protective measures; the patient should also be referred to a trained counsellor, who might be a nurse with special training. Clearly, effective counselling that helps a woman deal with the consequences of her test results could enhancing coping. In practice, while all hospitals did some counselling it was not systematic. Of the fourteen women tested at a hospital, only eight said they had been counselled; of these some received little information or the counselling was incomplete. Only a few patients who were counselled at a hospital seemed satisfied with the amount of information, while those counselled at Sikukuchwa were satisfied. Women of course told me what was important to them. Whether or not these points were the intended emphasis of the counselling, they indicate the messages that remained:

The doctor counselled me. She said when you're HIV positive, the signs are diarrhoea, coughing, and all the diseases. When you're HIV positive, you must eat good food and keep yourself clean. No more pregnancies, because you can easily affect AIDS, because you loose more blood. Use Durex during intercourses with husband. She told me you must come to Sikukuchwa and there you can earn money and you can talk with others. (Tessa, 23, married)

I was counselled at the hospital. They said so many people have the virus. (Chipo, 26, married)

Then the doctor asked me in a private counselling room and told me your husband is positive. The doctor comforted me and counselled me and said: you must come to terms with the fact that you're HIV positive. (Nyasha, 26, widowed/boyfriend)

Women were almost unanimous regarding care and counselling in clinics and hospitals: to be counselled you must be lucky.

In the clinics it's a bit bad, no encouragement. (focus group)

In the clinics they don't do pre-test and post-test counselling. They just tell you that you are HIV positive and you are going to have AIDS and die. (focus group)

In Harare Hospital they told me in the ward my child has AIDS and there were so many people in the ward and everyone was looking at me. They just say it as if they are telling you that you have cholera or flu. (focus group)

Interviewees sometimes heard their status (or that of their child) from the doctor and sometimes from a nurse. The ways they were told varied considerably, from just telling a woman she was HIV positive to full information and post-test counselling. Pre-test counselling was uncommon, even though good pre-test counselling means fewer problems in acceptance and coping with results. Only one woman explicitly mentioned pre-test counselling:

First she asked me whether I know there's a disease which is new, that cannot be cured, which is AIDS. So she asked me if she can test me and if I wanted to be told the results. (Ann, 23, single)

Whether information and counselling were given seemed highly dependent on the person conducting the bloodtest. It is possible there were simply not enough counsellors for the growing numbers of HIV patients. It is also true that in Shona culture it is unusual to bring bad news, although serious diseases should be revealed. HIV is a condition with a double face: a person looks healthy, yet it can take years for full-blown AIDS to appear. This makes it particularly difficult for doctors and nurses too to tell a woman she is HIV positive. On the other hand, four of the six who were not counselled were in the lowest income group. Lack of information might also be related to their educational level and that none spoke English, the language used in Zimbabwe for most leaflets about HIV/AIDS. Non-English speakers must depend mainly on oral information. As a result of all of these factors, HIV-positive persons often receive too little information about HIV/AIDS and how to protect themselves and those around them, and almost no attention to their psychosocial well being after the frightening news.

The woman just called me and told that I was positive. (Jackie, 31, divorced)

They only said you're HIV positive. I heard it from the radio what it meant. (Thandi, 41, single)

Did you know anything about this? Don't worry about it, he said. You're not dying, you can last for ten years, but don't forget that you're affected. You must behave yourself and you must eat good food. And if you want to continue with sex with your husband, you must use condoms to protect yourself, because your husband is seriously ill. (Barbara, 25, widowed)

They see themselves as if they will not get AIDS. They see themselves as superior. (focus group)

Although the words in the next to last example may have come from either the doctor or the woman herself, it does suggest doctors/counsellors may sometimes think and speak for their patients. They may project their own norms and morals onto HIV-positive people, with little empathy. Even people who seem to remain at ease are often sensitive and lonely in the face of such an illness, and can benefit from someone who takes their problems seriously. Unfortunately, however, the last two statements reflect the general attitude: HIV and AIDS are terrible, but only promiscuous people get them. The community indirectly blames those with HIV/AIDS; people do not perceive a threat to themselves. There is a strong division between those who are known by others to have HIV/AIDS and those who do not know their HIV status. This is a barrier to empathy – to understanding and tolerance. Fear, indifference and ignorance probably are behind these attitudes.

Referral to the Sikukuchwa project

Most government hospitals in Harare and some government clinics (located mainly in the high density areas of Harare city) cooperate with the Sikukuchwa project, and thus could have been expected to refer women to the project, though it would have been up to each woman to decide whether she wanted to come. However, only nine women who were tested at a hospital were directly referred to Sikukuchwa by the person who tested them. Others were referred later: five were actively traced by the Sikukuchwa HBC team and one was referred by another hospital. The health professionals in the clinic attended by two women referred women they suspected of being HIV positive to Sikukuchwa, probably because they had no test kits and not much experience in counselling and supporting people with HIV. However, no hospitals systematically referred women who tested HIV positive. As with counselling, referral appeared to depend on the willingness of the health professional, not on the kind of hospital. Too, women who did not speak English and were not counselled appeared even less likely to be referred to Sikukuchwa: their limited command of English may have prevented their finding and getting access to sources of support.

Health status

Table 2 outlines the stages in HIV infection used in this publication, which are of particular importance since the stage in which an HIV-positive woman finds herself may influence coping ability. Annex 1 describes the health status of each woman.

At the time they were interviewed, most women were fairly healthy. Two women were asymptomatic (Pretty and Helen, who doubted their diagnosis). In the majority, the disease had progressed; three had long-lasting swollen glands (PGL) and eight had HIV Related Diseases (HRD). Five had recovered from severe illnesses but some symptoms remained (ARC). One woman developed full-blown AIDS during the first weeks of my stay. Soon she stopped work at the cooperative and stayed in the Care Unit. Otherwise most women came to Sikukuchwa every day except when they or their child were sick. Although on average women had only known they were HIV positive for 14 months, for most the disease began earlier. While they did not clearly indicate when they thought the disease had started, most could specify symptoms and complaints they related to its onset – diarrhoea, fever, swollen glands behind ears and under arms,

Table 2   **Stages in the progression from HIV infection to full-blown AIDS**

Stage	Number of women[a]	Description
HIV infection (human immunodeficiency virus)		Initial infection with HIV.
Asymptomatic stage of HIV infection	2	Antibody tests are positive, but there are no apparent signs or symptoms of illness. This incubation period may last from a few months to a period of many years.
PGL (persistent generalized lymphadenopathy) HIV infection	3	Long-lasting swollen glands. This state may not occur; if it does, it may continue for months or years with no other symptoms of disease.
HRD (HIV Related Diseases)	8	Symptoms of disease increase because of damage to the immune system by HIV, but they are not life-threatening. Symptoms include diarrhoea, fever, vomiting, weight loss, coughing, Kaposi's sarcoma and skin problems. This period may continue for months or years.
ARC (AIDS-related complex)	5	Infections gradually become more serious and persistent, due to impaired immunity. More severe diseases such as tuberculosis, persistent cough, spreading sores, long-lasting diarrhoea, longlasting fever and cancers. Patients may recover from infections, but other symptoms remain.
Full-blown AIDS (acquired immune deficiency syndrome)	1	The terminal stage of HIV-infection. The immune system is severely weakened and cannot cope, so that life-threatening infections and cancers occur. The patient is terminally ill; death comes when an untreatable life-threatening condition develops. Life expectancy depends on the conditions that develop and the treatment available.

Source: Derived from the course of progression from HIV to AIDS described in Jackson, 1992 and from the AIDS Conference Report, 1992

[a] Number of women who were at this stage at the time they were interviewed

vomiting, loss of appetite, weight loss, coughing, TB, chest problems, skin problems (sores, ulcers, itching and skin rashes), Kaposi's sarcoma, Herpes Zoster. Many women tended to see any symptom as attributable to HIV/AIDS, even if it was not necessarily related – headache, worms, stomach pain, bodily weakness, feeling cold, breathing problems in summer, heavier monthly menstrual periods or no monthly periods. One reported something wrong with her eyes and another was epileptic.

Treatment-seeking behaviour

In Shona culture, serious or abnormal illness is caused by spirits, witchcraft or sorcery. Women at Sikukuchwa spoke of 'cultural' diseases – those that can be cured only by a traditional healer. Traditionally in Zimbabwean society, treatment for such illnesses is sought from a *n'anga* (traditional diviner-healer), whose main function is to communicate with the spirit world. The holistic approach of a *n'anga* helps determine and appease the ultimate spiritual cause of disease, to prevent further misfortune. Nowadays, more and more Shona rely on the proven success of Western medicine, especially for specific, clearly physical complaints. But Western medicinal treatment may be seen as alleviating symptoms while missing the underlying cause; thus one may consult a *n'anga* as well. Too, traditional healers are more successful than Western medicine in treating psychiatric cases or calming patients with terminal diseases, partly because they give more personal attention than is possible in a large, busy Western-style hospital (Bourdillon, 1987). In either case, the patient's change in attitude to sickness after the performance of appropriate rituals can be an important factor in the healing process (Bourdillon, 1987). But, although the effectiveness of suggestive therapy in some cases (such as opportunistic infections) must not be underestimated, a traditional healer cannot cure AIDS.

Initial treatment was usually sought from a *n'anga*, and some paid repeated visits. A visit was sometimes advised by the family, especially when they suspected a cultural disease. In the case of Thandi, her boyfriend married her, but her uncle (with whom she lived) asked for lobola (bride price). The man's family refused, but later they thought this was the cause of her child's death. All families who believed in cultural diseases and wanted the patient to consult a *n'anga* came from rural areas.

My young sister was worried: what is this for an incurable disease? She thought I had been bewitched by n'angas. She didn't laugh to me anymore [she was not nice to me]. *(Jackie, 31, divorced, ARC)*

The traditional healer said I was bewitched. Because my family didn't know much of it, they believed it. They thought it was a cultural disease. So it was very difficult for me to explain. (Tsitsi, 31, widowed, AIDS)

The death of my child was a cultural disease according to my boyfriend's father. He had cows and they [boyfriend's family and her uncle] *were fighting about the cows. Then a ghost came and took one of the kids. My boyfriend's father then gave my uncle the cows. (Thandi, 41, single, HRD)*

The relatives thought it was something traditional. They always say: a cultural disease, we should do something about it, because it is killing the whole family. So they're still buying cows, to pay going to the n'angas. Buying cows to kill for the ancestors, brewing beer. They were told in the hospital that my husband died of AIDS and that they should do everything with care, but they disagreed: one sister of your husband died and the other sister passed away two months ago. So you know we have to pray to our ancestors. They were really worried. They said the ancestors needed something. So they prepared a traditional cere-

mony, brewed beer and offered to the ancestors. In our culture they brew beer to respect our ancestors. (Nyasha, 26, widowed/boyfriend, PGL)

Nyasha made particularly clear what happens when the family suspects a cultural disease. From a traditional perspective this is rational. Subsequent deaths of family members break family ties and can be explained by bad spirits. Wife inheritance adds to the complexity: traditionally, when a man dies, his wife is inherited by his brother. When HIV/AIDS is involved, this may result in transmission to other family members, confirming the suspicion of bad influences from the spirits. But repeated visits to the *n'anga* can be expensive:

Oh, we had lots of money, we had property, we used to live in three rooms. We used to have a very big double bed and plenty of food. The n'anga was saying: you need this man [the n'anga], not modernity, I can cure the disease. Come, pay me 900 dollars and I heal that disease. We couldn't afford to pay, that's why my husband took the sewing machine. We were cheated. Now we are renting a very small room, because all the property was sold in order that my husband would be cured. We're living poor in fact through this, because we were ignorant of the virus. Now that I know I don't waste my time going to the n'angas who profit. (Nyasha)

When a person believes he is being troubled by spirits or other malign influences he cannot cope with, he consults a *n'anga* or diviner–healer. A herbalist, on the other hand, is a traditional healer specializing in the use of herbal remedies. Traditional medicine is sometime obtained directly at the market. It usually consists of a powder (made of roots, crushed branches or leaves, bark or herbs), dissolved in hot water and drunk by the patient (Mwanga et al., 1993). Sometimes the medicine is a ready-made drink, such as medicine claimed to be effective against STDs and AIDS. Unlike *n'angas*, who were mainly consulted by rural women and their families, herbalists were more often visited by urban women – those born and raised in Harare. Even if they disbelieved in *n'angas*, they still attempted to do something about their situation before or after unsatisfactory use of Western treatment. For those who first sought traditional treatment, when it became clear it could not cure AIDS women turned to Western medicine. Once at Sikukuchwa, the majority used hospital or clinic treatment and Western medicine alone, whether for self-medication or by prescription. This may have been because the majority were born in a city or had lived in Harare for years, making access easier. But also their urban basis may have lowered their confidence in traditional healers, and the influence of Sikukuchwa may have made them more sceptical. Usually, women said treatment provided relief for some opportunistic infections, complaints and symptoms, although this was often temporary, with complications re-occurring later.

I don't believe in n'angas. I don't think they can work. And also my father had no trust in traditional people. (Tessa, 23, married, ARC)

I go to the clinic or to the hospital, so that they can give me some medicines. (Ann, 23, single, HRD)

If I go to the doctor, I get a chemical, but they cannot help me. (Helen, 19, boyfriend, asymp)

Most went to Harare Hospital, Parirenyatwa Hospital or a local clinic for treatment. About half had a letter from Social Welfare allowing free treatment and medication. Both hospitals belong to the government and most patients are poor. Hospitals and clinics are rarely able to meet the demands on their facilities: queues at the main hospitals are always long. During my research all hospitals and clinics ran out of medicine, and Sikukuchwa had to provide them. Before coming to Sikukuchwa, six women living outside Harare sometimes travelled long distances to obtain treatment that was not available locally. Some (4) moved to live with a relative in town, to be nearer the hospital. One even came from Zambia, where hospitals were continually short of medicine. Judy took me to the rural area where she used to live:

Do you know why I left this place? Because I was HIV positive and had to go to the hospital each time. (Judy, 26, boyfriend, PGL)

I understood I couldn't stay in the rural area with this disease. So I said to my mother I had to do something in Harare. But I stayed there. I had to go to town, because with my illness you can't stay in the rural areas. (Tsitsi)

Although it was not common at Sikukuchwa, changes from Western to traditional treatment also occurred. The tensions and uncertainties of modern life readily provoke suspicions of invisible forces, especially witchcraft; few Shona can resist a traditional healer when things are going badly (Bourdillon, 1987). The n'anga provides a last resort when Western medicine has dismissed a case as hopeless, or has failed to cure it. Although all women realized that the sisters at Sikukuchwa disapproved, in times of crisis some sought traditional treatment, even when they had been at Sikukuchwa for a considerable time. This suggests the deep roots of belief in traditional treatment. During my stay, one woman went to a traditional healer and another to a herbalist. Pretty said she went to a herbalist to treat her stomach. Mary (not included in the sample) went to a n'anga when she had developed full-blown AIDS and was very ill. It was not clear whether this was to cure AIDS or to treat an opportunistic infection.

A third way of coping with disease today is faith healing, which is still growing in popularity throughout Zimbabwe and is often combined with Western treatment. This could involve prayer at home or active faith healing by prophets. The women who were Roman Catholic prayed in times of crisis. There are also the many independent Christian churches, which say they follow th e example of the Biblical Christ and his Apostles by healing all kinds of diseases through faith; they preach that using medicines of any kind displays a failure of faith and is wrong. To some extent the prophets and healers of these churches are replacing traditional healers.

In practice, Shona people may try all three types of healing in turn if they do not receive satisfaction. Although some maintain commitment to a Christian doctrine or way of life, theoretical beliefs are generally not as strong as the practical necessity of finding a solution in a crisis (Bourdillon, 1987). Because traditional healing has a very ambiguous position in Zimbabwe and not everyone wants to admit to visiting a traditional healer, practices were difficult to assess. The combination of Western medicine and prayer reflected the traditional beliefs mentioned earlier: Western medicine can alleviate symptoms and pain, but one must also combat the underlying cause. Most women (and/or their husbands) sought two or more types of healing. Some alternated among different types of healing as each in turn failed, spending large sums of money in search of a cure for AIDS:

My husband said the doctor hasn't treated him very well, so he went to the n'angas. He was given lots and lots of herbs to drink, to wash with, to ornament, but it wasn't of any help. Then he went back to do a new test again. And he was positive again. Then he said: no, they're cheating me and went to the prophets in churches. Every Sunday he was going to the church, so that the prophet could help him. But it was of no help. (Nyasha)

Most times I go to the clinic, otherwise I help myself at home. For example Herpes Zoster, it needs to bath. After sitting in the sun, those wounds will be biting me. With wounds I take tablets, because I can't be helped in the religious way. God will take some time to help me, God can help after a long time, not at that moment. So when I have a headache, I first take tablets and then I go praying. (Christine, 23, divorced, HRD)

When I've got pain in my chest, I go to Harare Hospital and I start praying with my rosary. (Noerine, 31, single, HRD)

Women who attended spirit-type churches sometimes made use of their claimed capacities of faith healing. Jackie belonged to the African Apostolic Church. Members are not allowed to use medicines, but faith healing was common:

I told the pastor the doctor informed me my blood was not good. He understood and comforted me, praying that God shall heal you and bringing your normal health back. I told him, for the pastor always wants to know about the virus. Then he prays for you to cast the virus. (Jackie)

In conclusion, many women at Sikukuchwa appeared to have actively sought treatment for their illness, whether from a traditional healer, a herbalist, Western treatment or faith healing. Some were consciously or unconsciously still seeking a cure. However, most women had stopped seeking and used only Western medicine to treat opportunistic infections. They turned to faith for their psychological health, which may have influenced their coping ability.

3 Communicating HIV status to others

Breaking the news of positive HIV status to a partner exerts pressure on the relationship; a woman must also choose whether and when to tell her family and/or wider social environment, and whom to tell. After examining the reactions anticipated from the social environment, this chapter explores the extent to which women at Sikukuchwa revealed their status. Personal evaluations of social relationships are then described for individual women (see Annex 1 for a summary). The degree of openness to partner, family, friends and community varied individually, but can be roughly classified as absolute secrecy, selective openness or openness mainly in AIDS Awareness Programmes. The actual response of the social environment is described in the third section. Finally, attitudes of the women at Sikukuchwa towards others with HIV/AIDS are discussed.

Anticipated reactions

I go on listening to the torture of my ears, the torture of my heart by those who have words as sharp as a razor. Words that eat into one like a bad disease which eats even into the bones of the victim....' (Chenjerai Hove, Bones, 1990, p. 14)

None of the women wanted to reveal their HIV status in their community; they feared discrimination, stigmatization and blame. However, the majority at least tried to discuss HIV/AIDS with others in general terms. This was an attempt to determine potential reactions and degree of acceptance. Some tried to increase others' awareness and educate them about HIV and AIDS.

I didn't tell anyone, but I have a friend with whom I discuss about the story of AIDS, not about myself. (Auxillia)

They don't ask, but I begin a story, then I say about AIDS and explain. Even other stories, but then they want to know how I know it. Then I say I read books and listen to the radio. (Tessa)

I tell other people: don't go outside and do something [have sex]. When you have a husband at home, don't go out for other friends, because you get positive. (Sarah)

I'm always telling people to use condoms to protect themselves. That's the best way. There's no other way to prevent AIDS. (Barbara)

In the focus group women indicated it is difficult to tell others because people know little about HIV/AIDS; media have made things much more difficult by portraying people with HIV or AIDS as dying victims and depicting women as sources of infection. Therefore community discrimination was expected, particularly for women. The woman who made the last statement here felt knowledge helps.

Because so many people think only prostitutes get infected, if you tell anyone they will think you have been promiscuous. So it's hard to tell anyone. You have to judge his reaction. (woman in focus group)

If I went on to tell the truth, they go around pointing she's got AIDS. They chase you away. You will feel isolated. I really don't trust that friend, sometimes she goes around gossiping. (Auxillia)

The people in my area don't understand how the disease is transmitted, they don't understand clearly about the disease. I think when I tell them, they think I transmit it to them and they don't want to come near me. (Judy, counsellor at the Home Based Care team of Sikukuchwa)

It's so difficult, it's not a story to tell next-door neighbours. It won't show a good picture, they will despise you, hate you, don't talk to you, gossip about you. It might help when people are educated and understand. But if they don't understand, it's of no use. (Chipo)

They don't like you when you tell. They think someone who is HIV positive is a spreader, even by greeting or something in the air. If you're sitting on the same seat in the bus, they think the disease can transfer. They would not react nice. (Tessa)

I don't want to tell, it's not good. Because in my location, they love me. If they would know they would say: that one is positive, better leave her alone. They don't want to stay with someone who is positive. When I had TB they avoided my house. (Sarah)

If I would tell anyone, they would run away. The people will not laugh with me, they will despise me, because they are not educated. They are still ignorant of the virus and therefore they are still afraid. (Jackie)

I'm afraid, because these African people, they don't know much about the disease. They don't accept it. They can run away from you. They can fear you and others go around and say: you know, she is HIV positive. When I'm in the last position, when I have full-blown AIDS, then the time is there to tell. It would only help if someone understands. (Ann, testifying in AIDS Awareness Programmes)

There are a few people who know much about HIV and AIDS.[1] So if you tell them, they will laugh [sympathize] with you. (woman in focus group)

Although Ann talked about ignorant African people, she had a relationship with a white man who deserted her, probably because he knew he was HIV positive and could not tell her. Notably, the women talked only about 'African people' in general; they seemed to overlook that though everyone is influenced by others, individuals can think for themselves. These women seemed to experience their communities as if they had to stand forward to be judged. Everyone, including those testifying in Awareness Programmes, believed it unwise to tell anyone in their direct social environment about a positive status. This made the strength of fear of discrimination clear. Some probably expected discrimination because they had seen it happening to others; others were influenced by the media or heard about it from others at Sikukuchwa, but the fear may have been greater than the actuality. Discrimination was the main reason, but many did not want to reveal their status because they thought it would not help; others would still not be able to assist – mainly with material, financial and practical support. No one was convinced that talking to other people might help psychologically or emotionally; Tessa mentioned the possibility, but it seemed of little importance. Their illness concepts had some influence here: HIV cannot be cured, so there is nothing other people can do to help.

When the results came out, she came and told me. I thought very horrible. I thought everybody would know the news. In the hospital they were talking and laughing. I thought they were talking about me and laughing about me. (Ann)

There's no help. They don't give me advice. If I tell my friend, she cannot give me advice. (Helen)

It does not help me. When I tell they understand, it's helpful to them, but not for me, because I'm already positive. It's of no help to tell anyone, because they cannot help you, except loving you. (Tessa)

Anticipated negative reactions and disbelief in the other people's ability (apart from women at Sikukuchwa) to provide support indicated women did not expect change in attitudes of others in the near future.[2] With these anticipations in mind, the third section of this chapter addresses actual community behaviours, seen through the eyes of the interviewees. They perceived reactions as discriminatory, but sometimes it was not clear why they thought so, since most people did not know their HIV status. Certainly there was discrimination, but the women seemed to try and affirm themselves; most never tried to talk with important others about their status. To some extent their own anxiety about discrimination and stigmatization appeared to be what stood in the way. Instead of stimulating each other to talk with people outside the project, women at Sikukuchwa often seemed to inhibit each other with negative stories, ideas and interpretations regarding probable responses from their communities.

Against this background, it must be emphasized that a woman must have great belief in herself and trust in others to have confidence that revealing a positive status will not harm a particular relationship. Further, not expecting to be offended by the attitudes and behaviours of the environment is one precondition for 'coming out' in this way. The construction and use of a social network is an expression of an individual's ability for control, self-efficacy[3] and social competence[4] (Schüssler, 1992) – factors which may influence coping strategies.

However, economic dependence on close relatives who could feel ashamed and hurt you, as well as prevailing social opinions, norms and values regarding sexual roles and relationships may make it particularly difficult for poorer women in Zimbabwe to reveal their status. Such potentially embarrassing news has considerable consequences for the personal well being of individual women. The following section describes whether and to what degree each of the women discussed HIV status with partner, family and close friends, and how they reacted.

Degrees of confidentiality: personal stories

> *The cloth on her head is torn and soiled with mud. She has carried the water-pot from the well for a long time. The cloth helps her head not to crack. There are other things she still has to carry. Things she does not know because they are things of the heart. She will carry them silently as she has done before, resolute. She feels the pain sink its jaws into her all the time. But she seems to take it all in one blow without telling too many people. (Chenjerai Hove, Bones, 1990, p. 15)*

Perceived potential for social support was likely to be influenced by women's illness concepts (Chapter 2) of their disease and by the anticipated stigma. Women had to evaluate their social relationships and determine the extent to which they could expect helpful social support if they revealed their status. Because of the continuing stigmatization, it was not surprising that no one was really open to other people about her status, although there was variation from absolute secrecy to selective openness with some relatives or friends. Three selectively open women who were also involved in AIDS Awareness Programmes were in a separate category, being more open to strangers. While convenient for purposes of description, these differences are artificial: women in this last group were also silent in their own communities; the division between absolute and selective secrecy is also more apparent than real, since a few women in the first group might have talked about their status if others had not done so in a negative way. Absolute secrecy, particularly for the first three women in this category (see below), is often the consequence of one-sided stories and gossip about them. For the other four in this category, silence seemed the result of good physical health. When confronted with their first symptoms or an opportunistic infection, they may begin to discuss HIV/AIDS. At the time, few women opened discussion with a partner: either they did not dare or because the partner had already deserted them. If they told anyone it was one or more family members; no one dared to reveal her status in the community. But sooner or later everyone reveals their status, or it is detected by others.

Absolute secrecy

Although Sikukuchwa encourages women to share their test results with at least one person outside the project, seven interviewees kept their status an absolute secret: one whose husband died of AIDS, two deserted by their partners when they fell ill, a married woman who talked only with her husband and three younger women who all had a boyfriend whom they told nothing. The first three were poor and living at Sikukuchwa, the married woman lived with her husband and the remaining three with one or more relatives. Two of this group had never had children; one lost her only child to AIDS. Two others had one child each, another two and the married woman three. 'Not telling' does not mean the topic never came up. A relative might suspect or someone else (for example, a doctor or nurse) might tell. For the first three women, the issue arose with relatives but women kept silent, anticipating a negative reaction. Relatives and friends of the other four did not suspect, probably because their health was good. The worst cases of discrimination were found in this category. All who lived at Sikukuchwa had problems with some or all family members, who knew or suspected they were HIV positive. They lived on a minimum incme and got no economic support from relatives – probably why they came to live at Sikukuchwa. Among them is Tsitsi, who moved to the Care Unit close to the beginning of the research project, because she had developed full-blown AIDS. Her husband had died earlier of the disease:

When I was in hospital, my father came once. Then he shouted that I had AIDS. Everyone could hear. He said: this is AIDS, she's a victim. With my brother and his wife I wasn't allowed to eat from the same plates, I got a plastic cup and plates and I had to sleep in the kitchen. I was not even allowed to play with the kids. When my mother found me, she took me to the rural area. Later, when I went to my aunt and uncle, they chased me away. That's how I came to Sikukuchwa.

Many women's relatives were afraid of contracting the virus and reacted by not touching anything belonging to them.[5] However, Tsitsi did not fear that her mother, who lived apart from her father, would react negatively. From the moment she knew she had AIDS, she wanted to tell her mother yet she found it difficult. She could just not start talking about it, because she did not want to hurt her mother. She said her mother had had a very difficult life too, and she felt very guilty. In June, her mother came to Sikukuchwa to care for Tsitsi. Tsitsi thought her mother suspected, but did not tell her herself:

I left my mother, because how can I confront her with her only daughter who becomes sicker and sicker and eventually dies. It's already difficult for her.... I don't know how to tell my mother. I can't explain myself. First she needs to come. I want my mother to know how I died. I want to tell her all my pro-blems.... I'm planning to tell my mother. My mother will not have big problems with it. Because the love I get from my mother is different from the love of my father and brothers. My mother won't gossip and go around, my mother can keep a secret.

I think my mother knows it, because she sent me here. She said I had to listen to that programme about Sikukuchwa. Why else would she do that.

Noerine, another woman staying at Sikukuchwa, had been deserted by her boyfriend when she had a blood test for HIV. As a commercial sex worker, she had heard about HIV and knew AIDS kills. She was with a man who was always sick (he had sores and venereal disease) and she was also sick, so she tried to talk with him:

With the man I was talking about our blood, because they had found something in his blood. I said: you can go everywhere, I don't know what you are doing. You're the one who is sick. No, he said, you are the one. My stomach was making strange noises, so he accused me of having the disease. I went to the hospital to test my blood. When they told me I've got the virus, they also said that I should tell it to my mother, brothers and sisters, but I did not want to.

It is not clear whether counsellors, doctors or nurses said Noerine had to reveal her status to her family, but it is clear that her personal situation and relationship with her family was not taken into account: procedures requiring permission of the patient before informing the family were not followed. Noerine's mother and oldest sister were told by nurses in the hospital without her permission, after which she was chased away from home:

My mother was very anxious and I was not allowed to cook anymore, my younger sister should do that. My mother gave me my own spoon and my own plates, and told everybody that it was from Noerine. They did the washing of all others together, but I had to do it on my own. They didn't want me, every time I touched things, they didn't want me anymore. I was crying there all the time. When they were told by the nurses in the hospital, they chased me away. She's still afraid now.... My mother started to talk with my younger brother and sister. Our lodgers also know, because my mother told them.... My brother and sister started to talk with me: Sissy, is it true what mother said – you've got HIV? They were all shocked about that.

This is just one of many examples of how activities called 'counselling' can produce more damage than support. This is not real counselling, because it does not start from the patient; others' morals and norms about the infection predominate. Health care workers and others should respect an HIV patient's right to have their status revealed only by themselves or at their request. Noerine had the good fortune that although contact with her mother deteriorated, her oldest sister helped her very much. But given the severe discrimination she had experienced, it is not surprising she did not want to tell anyone else.

My oldest sister doesn't care. She takes the same cup and we share the bathroom. We eat from the same plates with her husband, but he doesn't know. It's our private secret.... Because of that disease, my mother doesn't want to visit me. Sometimes I say: let's go to see her. It's my mother, I can't ignore to see her.

If it is not here in Zimbabwe, I can tell. If it is in Zimbabwe, I don't want. What about my face and my name? My older sister has got a television. Her husband always wants to see TV, I don't want him to know that I'm HIV positive. There's a programme about AIDS and he said: do you know that disease? I said: I don't want to talk about it. If you have sex with many boyfriends, he said. I said: I

*don't want. My sister would like me to stay with them, but her husband doesn't
like me.*

Joyce came to live at Sikukuchwa during my research period. She had been ill
and her husband had deserted her. She said her brother had hit her, but perhaps
she did not want to live with him because he suspected she was HIV positive.
His discrimination may have made her more unwilling to tell others, but above
all she did not do so because of her doctor's advice. A few years ago, advice
not to tell anyone your HIV status might have been useful, but this has had long-
term effects. Some women, like Joyce, are still basing their thoughts and
actions on what they were told in hospital. This can determine the subsequent
course of their lives, since it still affects what they expect from others (see
Anticipated reactions above). The first time in hospital is very important,
because it is the first confrontation with HIV. Health caregivers do not always
realize this. They need to deal with these issues very carefully, always emphasizing the need for individual choice based on ones' own situation and preferences, as put into words earlier by the women themselves (see *Testing and
counselling* in Chapter 2) and remembered by Joyce in this way:

*Long back the doctor told that you should keep it as a secret. When my hus-
band was ill, they also told me to keep it as a family secret. The doctor said:
the people would run away from you or despise you. That was information of
the doctor.... I'm afraid of being kept away, I will be discriminated or stigmatized. I want not anybody to know, because people will be pinpointing at me: she
has AIDS. So I just keep it as a secret. It's difficult, because when you tell one,
the whole location will know. You only can tell it when people are educated*
[well-informed about AIDS].

The women in the first three stories were all poor and economically dependent.
They could not choose to keep their status a secret; relatives had already found
out. Because they all had to leave their previous accommodations, their status
had direct financial consequences. But not all those who kept silent were very
poor. The other four who did not reveal their status were relatively better off.
One was married, with a working husband; one had income as a counsellor for
the Home Based Care team at Sikukuchwa. Both found it too painful to tell a
close relative, and expected discrimination. The other two women were in
denial and were more or less relying on relatives.

Auxillia was married and living with her husband. She started to work in the
Sikukuchwa cooperative while assumed to be HIV negative, but when their child
fell ill she and her husband were tested by one of the sisters; both appeared to
be positive. Although Auxillia indicated she would never reveal her HIV status
to anyone, at this point she had no choice, because Sr. T. asked she and her husband to come for the blood test and subsequently told them together. Compared
with others in this group, Auxillia could at least talk with her husband. She did
not tell her parents:

*We thought when we tell, it can pain them, affect them. Sometimes parents don't
understand and it can cause separation between relatives. I'm afraid to tell my*

parents, because they will be worried and when they see me complaining they will think I'm dying.

Because she was already employed at the cooperative, nobody would suspect her of being HIV positive even if they knew the target group of the project. However, since she had been trained to deal with people with HIV/AIDS and to be supportive, she might have been someone who could have revealed her HIV status. Also, others in her husband's family were HIV positive or had died of AIDS. Yet she and her husband kept their status a secret.

Two of my husband's family are also afflicted. He has a brother who is HIV positive. Last month he was discharged and we went to visit him in the rural areas and I read his card [medical card on which HIV was written]. It pains, because he's young and has two young children. To them we just say: God knows. Further, another brother's whole family died of AIDS. First the husband died in 1990. The child died six months ago and the wife last week. It's a problem, they left two other children and we don't have anything to help, since we're also struggling. My husband's sister agreed to keep the children, so she supports.

If I would do that [tell], it would give me bad thoughts, thinking all the time that people know that I'm positive.

The remaining three better-off women who did not reveal their HIV status were unmarried and living with relatives. They all had boyfriends but did not want to talk about their HIV status with anyone. Financially, Pretty and Helen were relying on their relatives; Judy was a counsellor for the Home Based Care team. Judy had never discussed her HIV status with her boyfriend, even though she apparently managed to use condoms with him. Further, she never told the relatives with whom she lived:

No, he doesn't know. It is too difficult. But I try to protect myself at the same time protecting others. I always use a condom.

I did not tell any relative. I will tell them, but not now. I will tell them when I feel like it. It's easier to tell persons you don't know.... I don't know how they could help me. I think there's nothing with which they can help me. There's no need to tell them, because I'm not sick. There's no need to share, I share with the people here [at Sikukuchwa].

Though Judy said it was easier to tell people she did not know personally, so far she had not revealed her status to anyone. However, she was a Home Based Care counsellor, visiting HIV-positive people and people with AIDS at home in the high-density suburbs in Harare where she lived. Although she had not told anyone, there was a clear risk for her that people would start talking about her work and might eventually suspect something.

Pretty was in denial. She kept her HIV status a secret not only from others, but also from herself. When she answered questions, she talked about others who were HIV positive, but not herself. Speaking of a relative who died of AIDS, she reacted empathetically yet neutrally. She also indicated she did not know whether people suspected why she went to Sikukuchwa:

My brother-in-law died, in 1991. For that moment I wasn't knowing of Sikukuchwa, otherwise I could tell Sr. T. and she could help. So I know about HIV and they haven't got a cure yet. So I feel real pain about him. His children can't go to school. His brother is now responsible for them. There was no reaction of me, because I was not knowing.

I don't think of that, just because some of the people don't think that I'm saying the truth, they think that I'm lying.... They behave in a different way. Some of the people, if you don't tell them the truth, they avoid you. But when I tell the truth, they are honest with me. They aren't hiding, because I show that I'm not afraid of anything. It will be open for everyone.

Yet Pretty did not tell anyone the truth. I could not assess whether she believed what she said or realized she was lying. Pretty also did not talk about her own HIV status to me, but she answered the question 'Do you do anything to prevent transmission of HIV to others' in the following way:

I don't move around, I don't have many boyfriends. And my boyfriend is a Christian, he doesn't move around. And he knows what HIV is, he struggles a lot.

Because asking for explanations during the interview did not clarify Pretty's answers, interpretation was difficult. Nor do I know for example whether she managed to use condoms with her boyfriend. During a visit to the countryside she told me her secret: she and her boyfriend were going to marry. During another visit, she expressed a wish for a child with him (see also *Consequences for reproduction* in Chapter 4). Pretty's vague statements suggest how much she may have struggled with her HIV status.

The third woman who kept silent was Helen. When I interviewed her, she had just come to Sikukuchwa and was still in the process of accepting her seropositive status (see also *Anticipated reactions* above). Although Helen was referred, the doctor did not tell her about Sikukuchwa. She clearly had difficulty deciding whether to tell her boyfriend. Without parents, having only a married sister who lived elsewhere and the working brother with whom she stayed, Helen could live relatively anonymously, more easily keeping her status a secret. Although she had no parents anymore, she knew why people do not tell them:

For that time I didn't know what Sikukuchwa was. I was not afraid, because I knew nothing. The moment I came here, I was getting afraid about what happened here. So it means I'm HIV positive!

I think in which way can I tell him? I still see him and we talk about it, but not about me. I say: if you get AIDS, you should do this and that. I give him advice. I told him: If you want to be safe, don't do sexual intercourse with many women. If you have one, stay with one. You can prevent with condoms. So you should prevent for your life. I tell him, but not direct. I feel guilty, when you conduct sex, he can get it. I use condoms. If you use them, you prevent pregnancy and the virus.

If you're HIV positive, you're nearly sure to die soon. So if you tell parents you're going to die. Parents don't read books, they don't know that.

A woman who hesitates to tell her HIV status is apt to experience the first reactions of relatives and boyfriend at the moment she becomes seriously ill. As this section shows, the reactions experienced may be quite severe, but not always as negative as interviewees had anticipated. Even if relationships with relatives have been bad for years, most seek contact again when a woman is seriously ill. Tsitsi told me about her father and brothers:

Now I'm ill and dying, they're all worried about me. My father rejected me and now he wants to see me, because that's our culture. I don't want them to bring me to the rural area and to arrange everything for me. I don't want to be buried. My father was not interested in me. I want to be burnt, so that nobody has to worry about me. They didn't do that during my life, so they don't need to do that when I'll die. (Tsitsi)

One exception regarding relatives was Mary. I spoke to her regularly but didn't interview her systematically (she is not included in the sample group). She had her own room of in the Care Unit, because no relative wanted to take care of her. Relatives came only once, to make arrangements for her children. Apparently they thought everything had been settled, so they would not be troubled by her spirit. Mary died as I was writing the research report at the end of 1993.

In summary, women in the 'absolute secrecy' category never told any relative they were HIV positive. (Judy and Tsitsi still intended to tell, respectively, a sister and mother, but immediately added they did not know how or when.) There were several reasons. Pretty and Helen did not accept their situation themselves; Auxillia did not tell her parents, not wanting to cause pain. Further, women are not used to talking with relatives about sex, and it is embarrassing to admit you have a sexual disease. This may also have been true for Judy, who said she did not know how to tell others. These four women maintained good contact with relatives, who did not know their HIV status and did not suspect, but this is apt to be a matter of time.

Again, not wanting to tell one's status may also be related to the taboo in Zimbabwe on discussing AIDS, and the fear of discrimination or stigmatization, even from relatives. For Tsitsi, Noerine and Joyce this fear was real, because of past experiences. Not telling others was a result of the negative reactions of relatives who did suspect, but silence did not have the desired effect. The three women had lived on minimum standards, not telling anyone; there is no way to know if they would have told someone had they not been living at Sikukuchwa. In this respect it created an artificial environment where they could feel safe talking about their positive status.

Selective openness

The reason for revealing one's HIV status is often security for the future, that is, ensuring someone will care for children or oneself. The person in whom women in this group confided was most often a mother or sister, presumably because they are closest, but also women are the carers. Nine women were open about their HIV status to some degree. Eight managed to reveal their status to one or more relatives; one woman told relatives and a friend. Three of these nine were married and one widowed by her husband's death of AIDS. The other five's relationships had broken up directly or indirectly due to AIDS – most had been deserted by partners. As a consequence, three lived on their own and two with parents. One had lost her only child, others all had two or more children. The three married women revealed their status to one or two close relatives, but did not discuss HIV much with their husbands.

Chipo's husband was in prison when she collected the test results of their child. They lived on their own; she told her sister because she felt very lonely, but also as a precaution. Chipo's sister reacted supportively and with empathy, which may have helped Chipo to feel less lonely and isolated:

I told her in case I would get ill, then my sister knows that the virus is active.

My sister also cried. And later we said: it's the role of God, let us know about this. At first she was really worried, but she comforted me that a lot of people have the disease. Last year my sister also said: you know, you're lucky that you know. Some people just die in doom, they are dying without knowing.

As will be seen in Chapter 5 (*Coping strategies*), in a sense HIV can give meaning to life and death; Christianity may support this. Relatives can help in this process, but also may be confused and feel insecure. When a woman thinks of revealing her status she knows there will be questions, which can put her under pressure. She may think she must know everything about the disease before deciding to tell. Moreover, she will be questioned about her most intimate personal life. A great deal of self-esteem and self-efficacy is needed to be able to tell others you are HIV positive. For example, to avoid being accused herself, Chipo had to explain to her younger sister that her husband used to go to commercial sex workers. Yet two brothers had already died of AIDS. Her words make clear how great the taboo on talk about AIDS can be; people therefore seem to die of nothing. The feeling of not being able to do something can lead to fatalism. However, this experience might have led Chipo to anticipate a positive reaction from her remaining brothers. Revealing her status might have helped to decrease the fear and helplessness her brothers had felt since the others died, but she expected the opposite and feared lack of understanding.

My younger sister was mostly the person who was worried about it. Because she knows that people who are always playing around get this disease, she asked: why did you get the virus whereas you have got only one partner?

My elder brother died in 1986. In the past, in the eighties, they didn't tell that a person had AIDS. They tied him in plastic and closed it. By the time we were going to see him in Beatrice Hospital, I was really worried, how he lost weight and became sick. For I had been seeing him for a long time, I really accepted it that AIDS was there. Those who didn't visit him, they didn't agree that it was AIDS. My younger brother died in 1992. My brothers knew that the young one had died of AIDS. They were told at the burial. They were afraid and worried, for the brother had already died, so they couldn't do anything.

Sarah was living with her husband and his parents. When she told him their child was HIV positive, he did not want to talk about it and said nothing was wrong. He was also sick, but for a long time he did not want an HIV test; perhaps he thought he had brought the disease (see also *Perceived cause of HIV infection* in Chapter 2), for he had girlfriends. As he became sicker, he wanted a blood test and became worried about Sarah and the child; this made her feel better. Sarah told her sister almost immediately when she heard her child was positive, because she could not cope with it emotionally. Her sister reacted with understanding, but her husband's sister did not. The husband's sister and Sarah suspected each other of being HIV positive, but did not talk about HIV. The last sections of this chapter show they were not exceptional.

My husband didn't react [about the child's illness]. *He said: go to Sikukuchwa, because I'm too ill. My husband is now not feeling well, he was a fat man.*

I told my sister everything, because it was hitting in my heart. I was so worried after the doctor said my child was positive, and I was positive. We started crying. My sister said: live alone, pray to God. She understands it now.

My husband's sister was afraid. I think she's HIV positive, but she doesn't want to know. When I didn't know that I was HIV positive, she said to me that I was positive. She laughed about me when I was getting ill and thin.

Tessa was very shy, lived with her husband and his parents, and probably did not talk with her husband about HIV. Her husband collected the test results for their child, but Tessa did not dare to collect her own results. I interviewed her just after a family death, when she did not want to talk about her mistakes with the rest of her family because it would pain them too much:

The sister of my sister-in-law had been ill and passed away last week with AIDS. Because she died, I didn't tell the rest of my relatives about myself being HIV positive. I only told my sister- and brother-in-law.

I want to tell my mother. Because she's the only one who takes care when I'm ill. My mother is the nearest person.

The three HIV-positive women who lived on their own – Thandi, Tendai and Jackie – also showed a degree of openness. All revealed their status to at least two people. They lived on a minimum income and had to pay their own rent. For example, at the end of a month Jackie often did not come to Sikukuchwa, because she had to find money for rent. Thandi was an older woman who had never married. Her boyfriend abandoned her when he was diagnosed HIV positive, without informing Thandi. When she learned her status she told her uncle and her son, because she could no longer cope economically. The relationship with her uncle was already bad, but became worse; her grown-up son reacted differently. She also feared loosing her lodging.

My uncle and me were teasing each other. Then I was angry and told my uncle and my son my partner was HIV positive and I, too. That they should care for a sick person and that I was in need of money, because of HIV. My uncle said: why don't you die, because you have AIDS and you give us a lot of problems, you're going to spread AIDS here. My son said: mother, you don't have to worry, because I read in the newspaper that an HIV-positive person needs good food, so that she can stay longer. Just because people will be afraid of me, they think they are also going to have HIV. And I am a lodger. When I tell I must move from my place, I won't have a place to stay....

Thandi lived with her uncle earlier, but had been on her own since 1986. Her financial dependence and a rented house were reasons for not revealing her status to anyone else. A home in Harare rarely provides the tenant with a sense of security. Tendai too thought she would lose her house if she revealed she had HIV:

Because if others know, they don't want to stay with me. The owner of the house would throw me out.

Tendai's husband had also deserted her when he heard he was HIV positive. She told her mother and brothers in case something happened to her. They worried a lot, because of other deaths:

My mother started to cry. I also have a brother and sister who had HIV. My brothers were also worried and said: we're all going to die of the same disease.... My brother died in 1989 and my sister in 1992. When he died we didn't know it was AIDS, only when we opened the box. At that time it wasn't allowed [to tell that a person had AIDS]. *When my brother died I was pregnant of my baby* [who later also died of AIDS]. *I was worried when I heard my brother died of AIDS. When my sister died, I hadn't seen her for a long time. She had a baby at that time and was sick, but we didn't know it was AIDS.*

When Jackie was ill, her boyfriend knew he was HIV positive, but could not cope with her disease and disappeared. They had discussed AIDS, but had never perceived their own risk:

My partner and I knew AIDS was there, but we never thought one of us could have the virus. My partner was the first one who had been told we were HIV positive, because he went to the hospital for the results of our kid. When I was ill after the death of the kid, I heard it myself that I was HIV positive. For I had been in hospital for a long time, he thought that I may die in his hands. He was afraid, so he deserted me. I don't know where he is.

Before living with her boyfriend Jackie had been married. After her divorce, she had sent her children to her mother in the rural area to save money. She told both her mother and her sister, as a precaution. For Jackie as for others, when counsellors explained the disease to relatives and they became familiar with the idea of living an HIV-positive person, many changed their behaviour, becoming more concerned and supportive.

I told my younger sister and my mother. I simply told that I had AIDS.... My young sister was worried: what is this for an incurable disease? She thought I had been bewitched by n'anga's. The first time she didn't laugh anymore, [before] she was always joking with me.

When my sister came here at Sikukuchwa, she was counselled by Sr. O. Then she started laughing with me again. After counselling we started reuniting again.... My mother didn't loose her love, she loved me so much and she's still loving me. She was really worried at first, but she has strengthened herself, because this is happening to people everywhere.

The last three women who were selectively open all lived with relatives. Two came to live with parents after a positive diagnosis. The other stayed with her husband's relatives after being widowed. 'Selective openness' is contiguous with the next category ('openness in AIDS Awareness Programmes'); the openness of Christine, Tambudzai and Barbara can be seen as overlapping these two categories. Christine was the only woman who dared (and had the chance, since most women had already been deserted by partners) to propose an HIV test to her husband when their child tested HIV positive:

I told my husband we had to go for a test, but he didn't want, so I went alone. Two months after the test I told my husband I was HIV positive. By that time he thought I already had AIDS, whereas on the card was written HIV. He said that we would no longer be lovers. He said: I can't stay with you no longer, you should go back to your parents. Because I know I'm not HIV positive, you're not the kind of wife I can stay with. He took off his clothes, because he was thinking I was going to pass him HIV.

Christine did go back to her parents. When her child got tuberculosis, people, among them her parents, were afraid and made her leave. After her first visit to Sikukuchwa she went back. Initially, Christine did not want to tell anyone.

The health inspectors went to our place to tell that we should go for TB testing. At that time people became afraid of my child. Then my parents started to chase me away and I came to Sikukuchwa.

My parents found out, because my baby was taking tablets, which changed the colour of the water. They cleaned the sink which had also been coloured and then they found out something was wrong. Then I decided to tell them the truth.... They answered that I didn't have to tell anyone, that would be the secret of the family.

Tambudzai was living in Zambia when she heard she was HIV positive. Because the health situation in Zambia is very bad, her aunt advised her to go back to Harare, where her parents lived. Her uncle accompanied her to Zimbabwe and told her parents:

I told my aunt secretly, when nobody was there. I was scared of my uncle, maybe he was going to shout at me.... My aunt told my uncle. They said: you're strong. Please appreciate what the doctors said. Don't go around with men.... My aunt said: no, it has already come, you should care for your body. We can't do anything, God knows, it can be cured. Maybe in future you will become alive. She said: go to Zimbabwe, there's Harare Hospital, where you will get treatment.

My uncle travelled with me to my parents and said I'm HIV positive.... My parents shouted to me: you've got AIDS. You bring AIDS here. My mother left me and went away.... So I told my sister: I've got HIV, not AIDS. I washed my clothes on my own. To my parents I just keep quiet, I don't talk, because they are old and problems can kill them.

Her brother and sister had died of AIDS, and the bad relationship with her parents may have affected her health.

My brother was working as a driver for my uncle in Zambia, but he's dead now. I don't know if he had AIDS, he was not tested, but he had diarrhoea, headache, cerebral malaria and was yellowed. He was hiding, he didn't tell me. And I have another sister who was having AIDS, I heard that in 1991, when she died. They were just following, first my sister, then my brother, then my child and now it's me, but I've been pushed by God. But my parents don't care about me. They want their children to die. If I knew that, I had not come here. I was just going to die in Zambia, like my brother did, he didn't want to come home.

I already have some problems like this, staying [i.e. given the way my parents are acting]. *Maybe in the future I can stay or God takes me, I don't know. When I'm going to stay I will suffer. My parents talk too much and they also shout. I don't know how I'm going to stay, how my future is.*

Tambudzai would have liked to talk about HIV with people who might understand, but had no one to talk with apart from those at Sikukuchwa. With a new boyfriend, however, she did not reveal her HIV status, but left him. She is an example of someone who has positive intentions, but finds it difficult to talk.

Like Christine and Sarah, Barbara opened a discussion on the HIV test herself:

I asked to go together to collect the results of the child, but he didn't want. Then I went on my own. I brought the letter to him and said it was from the doctor: I'm positive and my child also, I'm going to die. He didn't want to hear such nonsense. He said: you're not positive. They're telling you lies, you're fit and strong. But he knew he was positive and told me nothing. He said to the doctor: don't tell my wife I'm also positive.

In Zimbabwe, it is mainly men who are in denial. Women want to get tested and talk about their positive status, but fear of discrimination and rejection are obstacles. In general, women's weak position and dependence on partners leaves little space to insist on testing or on discussing HIV. A man who suspects something often leaves the home. When her husband went into hospital, Barbara felt she could not find the right way to tell her husband's mother that she and her husband were HIV positive, and asked the sister in charge to do so. Barbara told her friend last year. Once one person knows, it may be easier to tell others.

I was afraid to tell them. It was better that the sister-in-charge told in a correct way. I asked her: when my husband's mother comes for visiting hours, you must call her and tell my husband is positive.... My husband's mother reacted to my husband: you're giving me hard labour, when you die. What to do with the kids? You were on and on ill. She was afraid, thought that she could be affected herself. She gave me plates, I had to cook for myself. Sr. T., Sr. P. and Dr. R. told my husband's mother about HIV. After that she and some other relatives came in my home and asked me: what do you want to eat, do you feel better? They understood. Now they know, because I'm always talking to my husband's mother. She can always ask questions about the disease.

I told that friend I told you about. She's from school. She's the only one who knows about my illness. She was my best friend, so I could tell. She asked me: what is the disease of your husband? So I told her the story that he's HIV positive. And you, too? So you're HIV positive, she said, Come and sit here. She helped me. She always says it doesn't matter. She said: another person can die with a car. Maybe I'm also HIV positive. I've got a husband in my house. He can come across with another girl and bring the disease. Don't be afraid. She asked me: does your mother know? No, I said. She wants to help me by telling my mother. I agreed.... My friend told her mother. Now her mother wants to tell my mother. I said: if you want you can.

My friend wants to write my mother a letter. I said: if you want, you can. I think my mother will react, she will be shy, because I'm the first-born in my family. When somebody talks first with her, it's not so difficult anymore. I thought she will be afraid, because some people don't understand. She will think I'm going to die. I need something to explain, I know enough, but I can't.

She thought it might help a lot for her mother to know. She also talked about people who could help through organizations such as Social Welfare and some churches where she told some that she was positive. Still, she did not dare to tell others.

Yes, it could help. My mother would always know I'm sick. When she knows the reason she will not ask anymore. They can help me when I want something to eat. People who love me don't want me to think of it, so they can help me. Sometimes it would help in my mind. Sometimes, it doesn't, because people will laugh at me.

58

I don't want to tell others. If they know you are positive, they are going to chase you away. Like with Noerine. They chase you away, because they are afraid of us. So you must protect yourself. That's very bad. When we are affected we want to relax, but when they're always shouting....

In summary, except Tambudzai and Thandi, all women in this group maintained good contact with relatives whom they told about their status. The reactions of the relatives who were told suggest that fears of negative reactions were greater than their response justified. Although initial reactions could be harsh, generally the women were able to restore the relationship: relatives soon became supportive (mainly emotionally). The disease often clarified relationships with relatives. HIV/AIDS challenges a family because it concerns two very intimate issues: sexuality and death. This puts a lot of pressure on the family, but may bring about consideration of areas that have never been discussed before.

When a woman decided to tell someone, it was often a mother or sister. Barbara was the only one of 19 who told a friend. In Shona culture, as in many other African cultures, relationships between mother and daughter and among sisters are often very strong; these are the first people with whom a woman shares a problem. On the other hand, it can take a long time even to tell a mother, since closeness can make it difficult to cause such sorrow. Whether and how a woman would tell one or more relatives depended on her self-confidence and self-efficacy. For most women it was a matter of time and finding a way to tell. Here too, women often began to reveal their status when there was no choice: because relatives suspected, as a precaution, or simply because they could no longer cope on their own (psychologically or economically), perhaps when they became ill.

Openness in AIDS Awareness Programmes

No woman was really open about her HIV status. However, three testified in AIDS Awareness Programmes, telling many people in schools and factories they were HIV positive. Even so, they still said it was impossible to tell someone in their direct social environment. These three women were relatively well off, because they received income for testifying. One had no children, the others each had two. One was married and testified with her husband, one had been deserted by her partner before discovering she had HIV and the last was widowed but had a new boyfriend. None experienced negative reactions from close family; they seemed to manage quite successfully with discrimination and stigmatization in the community.

Not only Nyasha's husband but also two of his sisters died. His family saw it as a cultural disease:

After the burial ceremony I was told to stay in the rural area. Then I told them I was working in Harare and there was no need for me to stay there. Then I came back and they said: come to us, so you can be given another husband to keep you. Then I said: there's no use for another to keep me, as you know that my husband died of AIDS. They didn't agree and said this was a cultural disease.... Then I told the parents of my husband that his sister who passed away was also HIV positive and had been a commercial sex worker. Then I told that all the people know it is in the blood. They said: no, it has something to do with our culture. So you must be given to the brother of your husband.... I said: no, I don't want to be here with another husband, for my husband has passed away. I must stay alone. They didn't agree. They said: you just want to have sex with others. And then I said: no, you just come to my place and check I'm just staying alone with my two kids. They now agree that I must stay with my kids.

Nyasha also found it too difficult to tell her mother, who (as for Barbara) was told by an acquaintance, at Nyasha's request. Her mother reacted very supportively and they kept the secret together. Her mother was the only close person Nyasha told. With a new boyfriend, she did not dare to reveal it for fear of being left alone, although she suspected he was HIV positive as well (see also *Sexual relationships* in Chapter 4).

Ann had had two children with a white man who was often in South Africa. She no longer saw him and had begun to live with her mother. When she found out she was HIV positive, she felt very alone. She did not dare tell her mother, fearing discrimination or even being chased away. Eventually she did tell, mainly because she was economically dependent on her mother. Ann had anticipated her mother's reaction well, but realized she was afraid because she did not have much information. Although Ann seemed quite open in talking about HIV/AIDS, she did not raise the issue of her own infection with anybody else.

I found it very difficult to tell my mother, since I have nothing to help myself. I thought she would chase me away, although I have no money to rent something or to gather food for my children. To tell my mother took two months.... I only told at Christmas. I was trying to find a way to tell my mother about HIV. I had to talk about it. I was relying on her, had no money, no job. But to tell depends on the home situation, for some it is difficult, for others they can do.... At first it was very difficult. My mother reacted in a bad way, tried to chase me away. She was afraid to contact the virus and didn't want to play with the kids, even to eat from the same plate. That was because she hadn't much information about AIDS. Now sometimes we discuss, my family want to learn about it, even my mother.

If I had a special friend, I would tell her to be aware and to comfort me. Sometimes they can be supportive and feel sorry for you. And you can discuss with them to lighten your heart.

Marita and her husband were tested and told together when their first and only child died. Afterwards they talked about HIV/AIDS a lot with each other and started giving testimony in AIDS Awareness Programmes. She told a friend she met at a conference for HIV-positive people, and like Barbara she told Social Welfare as well as some churches. She said she could not tell her father and mother: it would hurt them too much, especially because she was the only child:

Because sometimes she [the friend] helps me. When I talked to her, she said to me: you must stay with your husband. When I told her she was very happy, because she's also HIV positive. She's feeling better now.

I didn't tell, because in my family I'm the only one. I think my mother will be very worried. So I don't tell my father and mother. It's very difficult. To tell my friends is much better, but to tell my mother... She will be shocked. I don't tell until God takes me. I've got no brothers and sisters and my parents are separated.

Especially when a woman is the eldest in her family or an only child, there is a great deal of pressure to fulfil parental wishes and expectations. Early in life she had to take responsibility for younger brothers and sisters as well as herself. This can make it even more difficult; she does not want to trouble her parents, often feeling guilty. This makes it safer to maintain secrecy towards parents.

Just as other women at Sikukuchwa, the three women in this category said it was very difficult to tell relatives or friends their HIV status; Nyasha and Ann each told one close relative, their mothers. Still, Nyasha, Ann and Marita testified to many in AIDS Awareness Programmes even though it involved the risk of being recognized in the street. They wanted to educate people and also received a little money. The risk of being recognized and gossiped about with people who knew them was not judged as very significant, because people they educated came from other suburbs. Sometimes they protected themselves, however, by using a false name. Talking in AIDS Awareness Programmes gave women a feeling they could do something to combat the epidemic, and may have helped themselves too, especially since they could speak openly.

I give my testimony in AIDS Awareness Campaigns to educate people in companies and schools. I want to let them know that HIV is there, especially Zimbabweans. I always like to tell others that they know, if you are HIV positive, it's not that you're going to die, you can still live. With people who need a lot of education, I give another name. You must talk wisely, you can see it at their faces when they don't understand. (Nyasha)

It helps, just because the more I talk, the more I get used to the virus. And I educate people through experiences. (Nyasha)

Nyasha and Ann had recently appeared on an UNICEF video about AIDS, broadcast by the Zimbabwean Broadcasting Cooperation. Marita and her husband had appeared in a short documentary about people with HIV and AIDS a few years ago, and had been interviewed by a magazine. As a result, anyone could have seen them. They seemed to realize the potential consequences:

I don't know if others know I'm HIV positive, they may keep it as a secret. But when they will publish the video, they will know. (Ann)

At the Salvation Army I tell testimonies. Some of the people see me on video and television. (Marita)

Still, even Marita had not talked to relatives and friends. The ambivalence and double standards about whom to tell and when, and what to say, was not limited to her; every woman had her own ideas and expectations.

Reactions experienced

From relatives

Although I had intended to interview family members and/or friends, this was rarely possible, simply because most had not told anyone in their immediate environment. I had to respect their privacy. Therefore the reactions and behaviours of relatives are described through the women's own eyes. It was remarkable how few of those they were close to were taken into confidence. They were afraid of discrimination and/or did not expect any help, even though as noted earlier in most cases people to whom they did reveal their status had apparently not discriminated in the way or to the extent anticipated. Seven of the nineteen had experienced some degree of discrimination. Of these, two relationships had been restored when the disease was explained to the relatives; two relationships had been bad even before the disease. Only three experienced severe discrimination from one or more relatives. It is worth noting that this happened when relatives suspected the woman might be HIV positive; we do not know what would have happened if the woman had been open, honest and able to give information about the disease.

It was even more remarkable how few women's families discussed HIV/AIDS in general, particularly since almost everyone knew someone who had died of AIDS. Auxillia, Pretty, Chipo, Sarah, Tessa, Tendai and Tambudzai all had one or more close relatives who died in this way, yet did not talk with family members. This safe secrecy could be related to cultural norms on informing the family about disease, but also revealing that a person had AIDS had formerly been legislatively prohibited; in any case the topic was avoided. Women who were the first in their families to become infected, like Tsitsi, Noerine, Joyce and Thandi, had to deal with more discrimination from family members than their partners or other women at Sikukuchwa. While negative attitudes could also have been because they were women or because some had been commercial sex workers, being the first to bring the news remains very important with respect to the reactions of relatives.

Community behaviour and perceived social support

Although the women told only close friends or relatives or no one at all, they thought others suspected them of being HIV positive. The reason was often that someone was knowledgeable about the disease:

I think my aunt knows, because she's working at the University Hospital as a nurse. She knows the symptoms. (Tessa)

Some who are educated [listen to the radio or watch TV] *suspect. But they compare with what they know. Because me and my husband are strong, they don't understand. So they believe our message that the child has got a big heart. (Chipo)*

They may know. If the relatives think of the child that died, they should know if they really understand AIDS. (Auxillia)

Many knew that Nyasha, Ann and Marita were HIV positive through their work in AIDS Awareness Campaigns. By 1993 Sikukuchwa as a whole was becoming well known, especially after a visit of the Minister of Health and Child Welfare, Dr. Stamps. As a unique project like Sikukuchwa expands, people will unavoidably come to know more about those who participate:

People think I'm positive, because they know I go to Sikukuchwa. They see the truck and saw it on television. They only think, they don't face me. I see it in their attitude. They don't say, because they think they are wrong. (Thandi)

Last week, when Dr. Stamps came, the people in my area saw me on television. They saw me with my boy and asked about my baby. My boy said to them it was Sikukuchwa, but those people don't know that the women there are ill. So I shouted at my boy very much and I said: you should tell them you go to school, not to Sikukuchwa. I said to the people that my boy is at school. They want to know, but I didn't tell them. I don't want somebody to ask whether I'm positive. (Sarah)

I'm always thinking of it. Because they always ask: what is the disease of your husband? Where are you going with your child in the morning? What's going on in your life? They know I can knit. And I come back with food. I told them I'm going to work in town. They're always ever asking me. They like to know. (Barbara)

Some people know about Sikukuchwa. A friend of my father's knows about Sikukuchwa. He asked my father what Sikukuchwa was: where's your daughter going? Suddenly the friend realized it's for HIV-positive people, but my father refused to tell. He didn't tell the truth. (Christine)

Sometimes the whole family maintained a stony silence, though the number of questions grew. Although people do ask questions, this in itself is not discrimination. But not answering may induce and stimulate uncertainty, and subsequently the fear that accompanies uncertainty. This allows stereotypes and misconceptions to arise or persist, increasing the potential stigma for HIV-positive women. Actual discrimination due to knowledge of a woman's positive status was difficult to assess, since most people officially knew nothing. At the time of the study, only Noerine had experienced serious discrimination from the community, after the family's lodgers were told by her mother. In most cases people suspected, but were not sure. Ten women experienced changes in behaviour mainly in a negative sense.

My mother told our lodgers. They said you're too fat now. When they see me they start changing their faces, even though they laugh, like they see another thing. They don't want to see me, because of that disease. They are afraid. If I go to the same toilet, they come with a sheet to clean it. (Noerine)

Some of the people say: Barbara is HIV positive, but she is fat, so she's not. They are confused. They are always asking: when you are HIV positive, why are you healthy? They think I'm cheating them. Some of them are very stupid, you know. (Barbara)

The behaviour of friends has changed, now they don't help me. When I want to borrow, they don't lend. When they see me, they gossip about me. Because of that illness. Long ago, they would give me money. When I want to sell the clothes of the cooperative, people don't want to buy, because they know it is from Sikukuchwa. (Tendai)

Though I didn't tell, people are afraid of me. They think I'm going to spread it to them. (Thandi)

Most people in the direct social environment were confused when women they suspected of being HIV positive looked healthy. This confusion appears quite normal, considering the reactions of people attending AIDS Awareness Programmes:

Some people don't believe, they expect someone thin. They don't know it goes in slow motion. They recognize me, especially schoolkids, on the street. They say: AIDS is there, just because I told them at their school. Nowadays I'm used, I don't mind. They just come and greet me. Some talk to me. They behave in a different way, some just come and greet you and ask for good advice, some talk to you, some want to pray with you. Some come and laugh and say: you've got the virus. Because they need to be educated, they don't know how to behave. (Nyasha)

When I talk to people, some are worried, because they don't understand. They don't believe that I'm HIV positive, because I've got power and I look smart. (Marita)

People find it interesting, but behind in the room there are always some men who laugh and deny AIDS. I laugh at them, because most times it are the men who transmit the disease. Those people want me to lead a normal life, to forget about AIDS, but mostly men want so. Some of the men really deny it's there. They say: you're lying. You try to make me afraid. I want to catch it.... But some feel sorry and want to change their behaviour. They are stable. (Ann)

A few women had lost contact with people in their area, mainly due to fear:

For I have been ill for a long time, so they are suspecting me of having AIDS. So they are a little bit scared of me. (Jackie)

Since my husband died, I haven't had anybody anymore visit me. I don't know why. Before I had. (Barbara)

Barbara probably did know why people did not come to her house, but this truth is not easy to acknowledge. She tried to cope very positively; acting in an offhand way may have been functional. If she had admitted to herself that people did not want to see her because of HIV, it might have caused a (re)lapse into negative feelings. She may have chosen to act strong, to enable her to care for her three children and maintain a stable life with her husband's parents.

Most women probably experienced changes in behaviour based on other people's suspicions. When behaviour did not change, women interviewees assumed it was because people did not suspect they were HIV positive. For example, the five who had managed to continue to live in their own homes and social environments (Sikukuchwa policy was to encourage this) were not yet sick, and were able to hide their daily trips to Sikukuchwa from most people:

There's no difference, because they don't suspect anything. (Judy)

Because they don't know I'm HIV positive. When they would know, they begin to change their minds. Because they are afraid. (Christine)

Two women who lived at Sikukuchwa expressed satisfaction and could not say much about changes in people's behaviour. Noerine had worked as a commercial sex worker, sleeping at markets and railway stations and looking very thin. Tambudzai too had sold sex; both were happy they no longer needed to do this:

They say I'm going to be strong. Some want to marry me. They say: you're keeping yourself so nice and clean. They're giving compliments. (Tambudzai)

You know, when I stayed in Mbare, I was slimming and slimming. The people said: oh, you have a disease. Then I went to Sikukuchwa and changed. Then I went to Mbare to show them. I prepared myself, I washed my body, I wore my glasses and went straight-away to Mbare. They were very surprised. (Noerine)

The fact that some women no longer had contact with the community or that behaviour towards them had changed could have more than one cause. Others could have changed due to knowing or suspecting a woman was HIV positive and fearing the disease. The woman herself could also have changed, due to her continual awareness of her HIV status and anticipation of discrimination. Most likely behavioural changes came from the interaction among these factors.

It seemed surprising that none of the group really wanted to reveal her status, even though many people suspected or knew it. even while people were gossiping[6] about them, they feared rejection, which may have made things worse since gossip lives on uncertainty. If the women had come out, there would have been no reason to gossip. The remaining problem would be fear, which causes the discrimination and stigmatization. The attitude of other people as perceived by the women (people pointing or laughing at them, or acting as if running away) was for the women the ultimate proof that it would be worse if they told. Yet the opposite might be more likely – that is, the possibility of explaining and educating about the disease, and perhaps eventually removing people's fears.

One could hope it would be easier for women like those at Sikukuchwa to reveal their HIV status in their communities if this were to become more routine and therefore more acceptable. If HIV-positive people were able to reveal their HIV status to each other, it could create opportunities to talk and support each other, and those who are at Sikukuchwa could then refer others. If organizations like Sikukuchwa were to broaden the current AIDS awareness programmes, not only providing more and better education in the community but also encouraging HIV-positive people to discuss HIV and AIDS with others with HIV/AIDS, it could have a 'snowball' effect.

Attitudes towards others with HIV or AIDS

It's better to tell someone who is also positive than to tell anyone else, because we have one thing in common. (woman in focus group)

This might suggest openness towards others with HIV/AIDS, but the opposite was true: apart from sharing experiences with others at Sikukuchwa, almost none of the women dared talk about HIV with someone they suspected or even knew to be HIV positive. Yet almost all recognized symptoms in others. Many women knew someone with HIV or AIDS personally; most immediately felt they had something in common, and were sympathetic. Seeing others in the same condition, they felt less alone.

I discover them, because some have Herpes Zoster, diarrhoea, wounds in mouth, lymphoids and are loosing weight. (Thandi)

I always diagnose people in busses. This one has glands, that one skin rashes. Also when they aren't tested I recognize them, because I've the knowledge. (Nyasha)

When I see them, I think these are my friends. I just want God to help them. They are the same as I am. I know that sick is a painful thing. I want them also to be strong. I also wanted the disease to take me away immediately, not to stay alive. (Tambudzai)

There's only one lady, who is staying in the rural areas, of whom I know she's HIV positive, through talking with her, seeing her and seeing the signs and symptoms of HIV.... I also thought this disease is almost everywhere. (Christine)

You can see many of them, especially here in Harare. In the rural areas there are less. Those in the rural areas come here for support. My neighbours, too. I just think we are the same, but I don't think they know I'm the one. (Tessa)

Most women reacted with empathy, and felt lucky to have Sikukuchwa:

I feel sorry for them, because they are at home, they have no one to tell. They think they're alone. Here at Sikukuchwa I feel free to tell about it and there are more. When a person would come here, I think she would feel the same. (Tendai)

There's a woman, who doesn't believe she's HIV positive. I feel sorry for her, because she has got a small child, she's not working and standing. Now she's pregnant again. (Judy)

I feel guilty when I know that this person is suffering with that disease. So I want to tell her: if you want to be safe or relax yourself, you should go to Sikukuchwa. Me, I'm lucky, because at Sikukuchwa there are some other people who are also HIV positive, but many people don't know Sikukuchwa. Like people in Chitungwiza, most of them don't know. (Helen)

Feeling this strong link with other presumed HIV-positive persons and their need for support, one might expect women at Sikukuchwa to do something to help. However, they did not dare say anything to those outside the project. This makes clear the strength of the taboo on talking about HIV/AIDS:

I just look and ignore. It's so difficult, people don't want to talk about it. Some are sex workers, they live on sexual money. (Joyce)

It's hard for me to tell about Sikukuchwa. Then they ask: how do you know I'm sick? There was a lady, a neighbour, who was also HIV positive. They took her home. I failed to tell her, I didn't know how to approach her. (Tendai)

I can't tell her that it's the virus. I don't know where to start. I feel pity for her, because she doesn't know. She's still a bit behind about the virus. (Jackie)

I did not tell that friend about Sikukuchwa, because she didn't tell me that she is HIV positive. She only told that she was ill. So if she doesn't want, I can't help. (Sarah)

I don't talk with them, I just look. Because if you talk to a person, he can beat you. Because he thinks: how can you tell me I'm HIV positive. (Helen)

I told Sr. P. about that lady. I can't tell her about HIV. Sr. P. has got the right to tell that lady. (Barbara)

Reasons for not talking about HIV/AIDS were diverse, but all were related to the difficulty of speaking openly. Only Nyasha and Judy tried to get people to a clinic or to Sikukuchwa (although Judy still did not reveal her own positive status). Nyasha talked to people she suspected of being positive. She was attempting a kind of AIDS Awareness on the street:

I know people, but they don't tell me. I see it at the symptoms they have. When I tell them they should go to the clinic, they ignore. (Judy)

Because I'm always talking, I know the people. I know many who have been tested, but don't accept it. They go to n'anga's and prophets. I always try to talk with them, for example a woman last week. She was complaining that she went to so many hospitals, but is not cured. Then I told about Sikukuchwa and she said: where is that place, because she wants to be cured. And then I said: when you meet other people who have the same as you, you can relax in fact. That's the cure. Then she laughed. They don't have someone to talk to, that's where our friendship starts. I don't mind to talk with someone with AIDS. I always talk with people who are despised by others. (Nyasha)

Nevertheless, it was remarkable that almost all of the women reacted to people with HIV/AIDS exactly as they perceived others reacting to them. Women at Sikukuchwa too gossiped about those with suspected HIV or AIDS; most did not talk to them. Several reasons were given: fear that the person would become angry or deny it – or ask how they knew! They could beat you or go to the police. As a result the women did not say anything – a missed opportunity on both sides.

4 Consequences of being HIV positive

For women at Sikukuchwa there were many consequences of being HIV positive. When HIV/AIDS is an issue, there is pressure on sexual relationships, and questions about practising safe sex. Further, HIV/AIDS influence decisions concerning pregnancy, as described in the third section of this chapter. The following sections discuss socioeconomic and psychosocial consequences of being HIV positive. The ways these are perceived may influence the choice of coping strategies.

Pressure on the relationship

If a woman who is positive does not show symptoms of HIV/AIDS, she may have a choice: will she tell her status or not? But if she is quite ill, she can hardly hide it. Not telling has the advantage that her husband or partner will not blame the woman, quarrel about it or disappear. The disadvantage is having to live with a haunting secret and the fear that he will find out, which (as discussed later in this chapter) may have considerable psychological and economic consequences. In the focus group discussion, the question 'Do you think it is your responsibility to tell your partner?' elicited the following replies:

It depends on the type of the partner.

Yes, it's my responsibility to tell my partner, but it's hard to tell. If the wife knows she's positive, she won't tell her husband, because she will be afraid of being told she is the one who brought it. And the husband will do the same.

It's very difficult. But it's easier when you have a child. Because then the doctor says we have to come for a test together, because the child is positive. If there's a child you know how to tell.

When the husband knows he's HIV positive, he will not tell us, he keeps it for himself.

When my husband knew it, he only said we should use condoms.

But as a woman to tell your partner, is impossible.

These remarks illustrate how much the lives of Zimbabwean women, and the choices they make, depend on the husband or partner. Her behaviour and what a woman can say or not largely depend on him; the husband always has the limiting role. A woman often knows exactly how far she can challenge her partner before he gets angry, beats her or goes away. In the eyes of the women at Sikukuchwa, few men react with understanding and want to sit down to discuss the problem.

AIDS often put great pressure on a relationship. Almost none of the women had explicitly discussed HIV with a partner. When they dared to tell, husbands or partners often did not want a blood test, denied that AIDS was there, were afraid of being HIV positive themselves or afraid of having to care for a sick person. As a result, men did not want to admit their own HIV status and/or immediately ran away: seven of 19 relationships had ended directly or indirectly due to AIDS. This had happened to three of the five divorced women. One was left when she was ill (Joyce, see Chapter 3, *Absolute secrecy*), one when she told her husband she was HIV positive (Christine, see *Selective openness*, Chapter 3) and one because the husband knew he was positive (Tendai, see *Perceived cause of HIV infection*, Chapter 2). Further, three of the nine who had a boyfriend before coming to Sikukuchwa had been deserted, probably because the men knew they were HIV positive and left before the women were tested (see further Noerine, *Absolute secrecy*, Chapter 3, Thandi and Jackie in Chapter 3, *Selective openness*). Lastly, one of these nine women, Tambudzai, broke up with her boyfriend herself. He wanted to marry her, but she refused. She told him she was too sick.

I had been ill for a long time. When I was ill, he ran away and stayed with someone else. (Joyce, 29, divorced)

Before the second child got ill, the father went to Parirenyatwa [hospital in Harare] and heard he was positive. He never told me, but ran away, because he was afraid. When the child would fall ill, he would have to do another test and I would find out. He now lives with another woman, but he's ill and wants to go back to me. But I don't want. (Thandi, 41, single)

Of the seven women whose relationships ended due to AIDS, only one (Christine) had proposed an HIV test to her husband, because their child appeared to be HIV positive. Others did not dare talk about HIV/AIDS or had no chance – the partner had already left. It was notable that partners typically left only after an event such as the illness of the woman, or in one case (Thandi) a child. When a woman's husband had full-blown AIDS, she cared for him until he died, but the opposite was not true: women were often deserted by partners.

Talking about this subject was no less difficult for the five married couples who were still together. They all learned they were HIV positive when a child fell ill. Only two couples (including Auxillia and Marita) were tested and told together about their HIV status; three couples still did not know their results at the time of the interviews, though two had (positive) results for their child and all women had been referred to Sikukuchwa. One couple (Chipo) was tested together, but said they did not have their results, one (Tessa) did not dare collect test results and one (Sarah) said she was told only that she had TB, nothing about HIV; her husband did not want to collect his results. People do not collect their test results for various reasons, among which fear may predominate. Also, there is often a two-week wait before results can be collected; by assuming education and counselling can wait until results are picked up, hospitals miss the best opportunity for, since this may never happen. Even if a woman wants to know her status, she leaves the initiative to her husband: asking may put her marriage at risk. It seems unlikely that couples who did not know their results had talked much about HIV and AIDS; their tests had been conducted more than half a year earlier. This indicates how difficult it was to talk about the illness in all relationships.

Three women had been widowed when a husband died of AIDS. The consequences of disease and death were considerable. Just as when a partner left, the woman was confronted with new problems: how to get support? What about my children? These problems often forced her back to her parents. Most women who came to Sikukuchwa were attempting to avoid this.

My husband was always sick. I cared for him for three years. (Barbara, 25, widowed)

It changed my whole life. My life is miserable. Only when my husband was alive, I enjoyed my life. But then God took him from me. Why did God take him? And then I had one child left whom I could love, but he also died. (Tsitsi, 31, widowed)

When my husband died, I was really worried that there was no one to look after my kids and that he had left the virus with us. I was really alone, there was nowhere I was going to, in the rural areas I was going to die. And the family wanted to give me another husband, so it was difficult for me. (Nyasha, 26, widowed/boyfriend)

Sexual relationships

I didn't tell him I'm HIV positive. But I suspect he's HIV positive, too. I always use condoms or try not to have sex. But it's difficult for me, as a lady, whose husband died. Do you know that scientifically, can I have feelings [sexual desires] sometimes? (Nyasha, 26, widowed/boyfriend)

Women have various reasons for wanting to have sex: making love as part of a long-term relationship; sex for pleasure; to become pregnant; to gain affection and emotional closeness; as a duty, service or profession; to secure financial support to survive; to obtain favours; or to achieve a socially acceptable position (Berer and Ray, 1993). Power imbalances between men and women make for a lack of safety in sexual relationships; HIV/AIDS has become an additional threat.

At the time of the interviews, four women had boyfriends (Pretty, Helen, Nyasha and Judy). All four had sexual intercourse with the boyfriends, so without condoms there was a real fear of infecting them. The women, however, also feared their partner would run away if he knew. They were not ill and did not say they worked at Sikukuchwa, so they could hide their secret. Moreover, two were in denial (Pretty and Helen) – perhaps the reason they did not tell. While none managed to talk about it, one tried (Helen, see *Absolute secrecy*, Chapter

3). However, they all said they protected themselves and their boyfriend against HIV infection by using condoms. Their partner's acceptance of this suggests the empowerment of the four women. A Zimbabwean woman who proposes the use of condoms is often accused of unfaithfulness or prostitution. Women need self-efficacy and competence to even open a discussion on the issue of safe sex. It is likely that the women did do this, although it may be that they sought out men who brought it up, perhaps because they were HIV positive themselves or because they really saw the necessity to use condoms. The five married women still had sexual intercourse as well. Four couples protected themselves by using condoms during intercourse, of whom two couples (Sarah and Tessa) said they did not know their results of the HIV test, while two (Marita and Auxillia) knew they were HIV positive:

I use condoms, I don't want to go for another man, because then I get pro-blems. I live only with one man. (Sarah, 23, married)

It's very easy, it's just me and my husband, so we use condoms. We get them at Pari [Parirenyatwa hospital] *and the Red Cross. (Marita, 22, married)*

We use condoms, we get them from Sr. P. I was using pills, but I had no money to buy them. My husband was not working that time. Sometimes you don't have money yourself. So when I ask for money and he says: buy meat, what can you do? (Tessa, 23, married)

Sometimes, particularly since the Ministry of Health had ceased distributing condoms for free, there was literally a choice between food and contraceptives – hardly a real choice. Condoms were, however, again available at cost price.

Chipo did not know her results either, but she did not do anything that would prevent transmission. The other ten women, although not having sex is hardly imaginable in Zimbabwean culture, preferred this option and abstained.

We still have sexual intercourse, but we use precaution, feminine tablets. (Chipo, 26, married)

I don't think I'm going to do such a thing, otherwise I'm going to spread. I have to stay away from men and boyfriends. (Christine, 23, divorced)

I'm now staying as a nun-person. I'm afraid of men, I can't share sex with any man. I think when I share sex with many men, I will destroy many lives, I will infect many others. (Thandi, 41, single)

I give my policy of no more sex. I'm not going around with others. But to the others I say: use condoms. But they can burst and some don't use them in the right way, so it needs faithfulness. (Ann, 23, single)

At the moment I have no sex, because I'm still crying for my husband. I can't. (Barbara, 25, widowed)

Consequences for reproduction

How can a man marry and then sleep with his wife for so long without making her pregnant? Poverty started fighting me long ago, Marita. Do you not remember the days all people came to try to take you away to a medicine man to see why you could not nourish the seed I planted in you? The woman's womb is dry, she ate all her eggs. The woman should give the man a chance, let him have another woman, then we will see if the nest continues to be empty. We cannot allow a name to die. The man cannot be buried with a rat. Yes, the man would have to be buried with a rat on his side if he dies without a child. Shame. That will be the end of the name. Childlessness is a sign of evil in the house. (Chenjerai Hove, Bones, 1990, p. 27)

As in most African countries, having children is very important to a woman in Zimbabwe. Her status comes from bearing a child, especially when it happens to be a son. When the first child is born, her first name becomes Amai... (adding the name of the child) – the mother of.... If her son or daughter has a child, she becomes Ambuya...., grandmother of.... Women's names thus always express their relationship to their children. When people call a woman Amai or Ambuya, it is an expression of respect. Addressing her by her own name expresses disrespect – or that she has no children. One doctor said:

African women are born to have children. According to the culture do not become an ancestor if you don't have children. Every woman wants children. Because the transmission is not 100%, many still want to have more children, even when two have died. What is important is for people to see that the woman is pregnant, even if the baby is HIV positive. (Paediatrician Parirenyatwa Hospital, personal communication)

However, 15 of 19 women already had children; few wanted more.

Because I had three who died and now I have three left. I don't hope to have another child, because when I give birth, the baby is going to die. (Auxillia, 39, married, 3 children, 3 died)

Two is enough. When I'm pregnant, I'm dying. When the doctor explained that a person who is positive should not get pregnant, we didn't want to know about children again. (Sarah, 23, married, 2 children)

I've got a boy and a girl and I'm carrying the virus. When I see the mothers, it's a hard time, when an innocent child is born [who might get the disease]. *It's really terrible and paining. (Ann, 23, single, 2 children)*

Because I'm facing a lot of problems. I have heard of it that once you become pregnant when you're HIV positive, you get the symptoms. And also the kids can become sick, so that you have no time to rest. You will always be rushing to hospital for the kids and yourself. (Christine, 23, divorced, 2 children)

Ten is enough. In hospital they told I was tired of having children, that's why my child is sick. (Tendai, 42, divorced, 9 children, 1 died)

Women are generally told at the hospital not to have more children. Health carers often feel they know best and do not allow women and their partners to decide for themselves. Women at Sikukuchwa often mentioned such moralizing attitudes, but clearly some of the women above had made a conscious choice for themselves, without judging others who may wish for more children.

The majority of women had been pregnant since having HIV; many had experienced severe problems and had borne an HIV-positive baby. Though not all had been tested, most younger children at Sikukuchwa were ill time and again, and were probably HIV positive. Older children were likely to be free of HIV, but apt to become orphans within a few years.

Tessa gave a vague answer to the question of whether she wanted to have more children because she appeared to be pregnant.

But it can be a mistake. You can get pregnant, like now. I am not settled, I am not feeling all right. I am thinking of myself, I can die when I deliver. My body is all right. I'm about six months pregnant. My husband doesn't know and he doesn't see it. He does not want more children, because of ESAP [economic hardship due to the Economical Structural Adjustment Programme]. *I'm just keeping quiet, until the days are full. (Tessa, 23, married, 2 children)*

Tessa knew exactly how to protect herself, so I asked how that happened. She laughed, seeming to accept her situation with ease. Later she hinted at worries. In Zimbabwe, abortion is illegal and difficult to carry out; women like Tessa do not have a choice. Health professionals, family and the community may express concern for her welfare and that of her child, but she may also face fear, disapproval and rejection by some (Berer and Ray, 1993). Women's opinions on number of children are strongly influenced by prevailing social norms and values, including those of their husbands and the government. In the past most had six or more, like Auxillia and Tendai, the oldest women participating at Sikukuchwa. At present, having fewer children is encouraged; most limit the number for financial reasons. But for most women two children are the minimum for status as mother and to confirm the bond with a partner.

Four HIV-positive women, of whom three were childless, expressed an intention or a wish for a child. Three were very young; the fact that they were not yet mothers was very important, in spite of their positive status. Tambudzai and Marita wanted children only if they became healthier; each had lost a baby to AIDS, which may have influenced them. Helen and Pretty definitely wanted children.

Unless the doctors say I'm okay. I don't know if we, HIV-positive women, must bear children. The doctor said when I get one, it will die. I have to follow the doctor's advice, not doing it for myself. (Tambudzai, 26, single, 1 child died)

I want to have a child. It's good to have your own child. Even one. My boyfriend also wants to have children. We are not talking about it. He talks to friends and his friends told me. When I've got a child without HIV, *then I will be happy. I want to try. (Helen, 19, boyfriend, no children)*

Yes, only one. I have one, so I want to have another one. I want to have two kids, not more, because cost of living is now very difficult for everyone. When I marry, I want to become pregnant at any time. (Pretty, 21, divorced/boyfriend, 1 child)

Notably, Pretty and Helen were also the two who denied their status. Perhaps coping through denial opens a possibility to choose to have children. On the other hand, a strong wish for children could cause women to deal with their positive status as if it were not true. Moreover, each had a boyfriend; this also might promote a strong desire for a child: Pretty explained to me that you cannot stay together as man and woman without having at least one child.

Other women, most of whom already had had at least one child, appeared to have fewer problems with the knowledge that becoming pregnant would be a risk. Compared to childless women, their families and social environments had far less strong expectations that they become mothers. Noerine and Tsitsi, on the other hand, said clearly that they did not want babies even though they were childless. Tsitsi had logical reasons; she then had full-blown AIDS and only wanted to die. After her husband died, she had never considered having children. Noerine, however, expressed the importance for women of becoming mothers:

The disease influenced my life very much. I have no baby, I have no anything. When I would have a child... [showing me some baby clothes she kept in her room] (Noerine, 31, single, no children)

At Sikukuchwa, the idea that women should make their own reproductive choices and should respect each others, choices was emphasized. Whether or not to have children was also often discussed in the support group. While preparing for the focus group discussion, Ann (treasurer of the group) and Nyasha (chairperson) said:

It's your own choice. You know the child can be positive and can be sick each time, or can be negative, but then you have to find a carer. And for yourself, for your own health it is risky to have a pregnancy again, because you loose blood and it can stimulate the virus. (Ann)

You know it's a chance fifty-fifty. So some decide to take the chance. Or to have two children, so there's a big chance that one is healthy. (Nyasha, 26, widowed/ boyfriend, 2 children)

Socioeconomic consequences

Most women faced direct socioeconomic consequences when they, their husbands or their children became ill. Direct impacts were generally a loss of income and basic shelter (in the quotations, e.c. stands for economic category; see Table 1):

It really affected. Firstly, when the child was ill, we wasted much money trying to get help from the doctors, but we didn't get help. The other change is that I was staying in the rural area. When we heard we were HIV-positive, we stopped staying at home. (Auxillia, 39, married, e.c. 5)

When I became ill, nothing went okay. I was unable to do something [to work]. And the illness took my husband. Much property has been sold to get money for living. (Nyasha, 26, widowed/boyfriend, e.c. 4)

When I was staying in Zambia, they [aunt and uncle] kept me nicely as a patient, though they had shortages of medicines. Here my parents are not nice for their children, that's the way they are. In Zambia, you can work. Here if you sell things, the police catch you. It's too difficult. (Tambudzai, 26, single, e.c. 2)

Others lived with the threat of losing their homes (Thandi, Tendai and Jackie) or jobs: keeping silent about one's status was sometimes necessary. In the long term, HIV and AIDS drained women of resources and their standard of living declined. Some husbands died, others deserted. As a result, income from the partner disappeared. Moreover, most had children to care for. In addition to the usual expenses, they had to find extra money for medical treatment; but due to their own illness or time spent caring for sick children or a husband they lacked time to earn money. Loss of income and a lower standard of living made it necessary to set priorities.

I used to sell some fruits, to get income, buy food for the kid. Nowadays I can't do anything, just sitting, no one can give me money, because my husband ran away from me. (Joyce, 29, divorced, e.c. 1)

Long back I used to do things on my own, working. Now I'm just sitting, waiting for money to be given. The illness disturbed me working and my health. I can't do things by myself, I'm always ill. I'm worried, because before I was ill I went to many countries, Botswana, South Africa. Now I wanted to go to Zambia, but I'm not fit. (Jackie, 31, divorced, e.c. 1)

I might be facing a problem when one of my children gets sick. Then I have to give money for the clinic. There will be no soap, no salt in the house. I have to use the money I had planned to use for food. (Christine, 23, divorced, e.c. 3)

In the first days, I was worried very much. I was leading a very difficult life. When you've got AIDS, you should not work hard, because you become tired. But I hadn't enough. (Ann, 23, single, e.c. 4)

My own problem is that I don't have a regular income. Sometimes I want to go to the clinic, but we don't have money. (Judy, 26, e.c. 4, said before she became a paid counsellor on the Home Based Care team)

Many of the options these women might otherwise chose would be a threat to their health and that of their children. In the end, minimum food intake, working too hard and lack of medical care will work against their survival (Barnett and Blaikie, 1992). Only three of 19 women said their life had not changed much due to being HIV positive:

There's nothing changed, because I was always sick. There are so many changes in my life, the illness is just one thing. (Tendai, 42, divorced, e.c. 1)

Only because my husband died, it changed, I mean for food. But not many things changed since I was diagnosed. (Barbara, 25, widowed, e.c. 3)

I didn't see the change, from I was healthy till I was HIV positive. It is just the same. It's just a disease like other diseases. (Tessa, 23, married, e.c. 5)

So for some, HIV is just one life event among others. Especially when it is necessary to work hard to obtain food and money for the day, long-term problems may fade into the background. HIV becomes more noticeable only when someone is especially ill and time and treatment costs interfere with earning money. Being able to pay for basic needs was a reason to feel happy and worry less about one's disease:

When I've got everything, no problems, life will be good. When everything is going okay, money, food, kids are okay, when I'm not sick. I always want to live happy, but that's impossible. (Nyasha)

Sometimes at Sikukuchwa they give me money, millet meal, clothes. So I'm not worried. (Marita, 22, married, e.c. 5)

I will be happy when I'm feeling better and have money to pay the rent. Especially this month I'm happy, because I sold the bedspread and I got money from the cooperative. (Jackie)

The health care system in Harare is relatively advanced in comparison to many other African countries and regions; many diseases that previously caused early death can now be cured, and belief in Western medicine is strong. Therefore as in Western countries, experiencing the limits of health care and accepting a disease as incurable is very difficult. This may have been the reason most women considered HIV/AIDS the most terrible disease possible.

Although many people in Zimbabwe face similar socioeconomic problems, they are more substantial for a woman who is HIV-positive. It takes time and money to care for her own physical and mental health and that of her children, but she needs this time and money to make ends meet. In many cases (10), there was no family member to help. The other nine women received one or more types of support from one or more relatives: school fees, money for school uniforms and exams, childcare, food, care when sick, clothes, medicine, other money for children, soap, rent, a brothers' loaned bicycle, blankets or cash. For most, economic support had not changed when they became ill; relatives could not afford more, or they did not know she was HIV-positive.

Socioeconomic consequences of the disease were great for all women, but affected women in the two lowest economic categories (see Table 1) most: almost all were single and living on their own. They were not supported by relatives and lived primarily on support from government Social Welfare, the church and/or Sikukuchwa. Regarding their HIV-status, they were absolutely closed or open only to some degree with relatives or others. All women who received support from Social Welfare are apt to have had a notation on their cards that they were HIV positive, and thus would have received money and free medication. However, most did not tell me whether welfare staff knew they were positive. Only Barbara and Marita said they had told Social Welfare; they were also the only two who said it was not a problem to state their status at Social Welfare or churches. On the contrary, they thought it helped. Marita and Barbara probably felt better able to cope with potential negative reactions from the community than others. Barbara's strategy was to try and take no notice.

When I go to Social Welfare I show my card, so they know that I'm HIV positive and I have no husband. Even in the church they know I'm positive and I need help. They know the disease wants to eat [requires money for food and medical care]. *(Barbara)*

I need especially money to pay the rent. Sometimes I go to Social Welfare. Sometimes they have money, but not every month. The Salvation Army Church also helps me, they give some clothes. So I'm happy when I talk about HIV to someone. (Marita)

I don't notice that. When I come home I go directly into my house, I don't see them. (Barbara)

For these two, the advantage of telling was greater than the disadvantage of possible discrimination. As a result, both received more support and were in a relatively better-off economic category. Ironically, some really do earn or receive money by displaying their positive status; this practice may cause serious damage to others with HIV, a problem funding organizations are not always aware of.[1]

Psychosocial consequences

For women's psychological health, an important consequence of being HIV positive seemed to be the uncertainty about what would happen in the near future, including the on-going threat of developing full-blown AIDS. Recurring symptoms such as swollen glands, diarrhoea, fever and sores, which caused women to go to a hospital or clinic, were constant reminders:

If you become sick, you will think that's it. I'm now dying. (support group)

I'm thinking about it, because it is difficult for you knowing you're going to die before you're old. You can die any time, so it's difficult not to think each day. And my child is ill every day, that's something that can affect me. For myself, I'm not worried too much, but when it's this child, the first born, it affects me too much. The first born is more important, especially when it's a boy. (Tessa, 23, married, 2 children)

At the present moment I feel a little bit sad, because of my throat. I think then: I might get full-blown AIDS. You never know. (Nyasha, 26, widowed/boyfriend, 2 children)

When things come, when my child is ill, I think: oh, maybe it has come to the point. (Ann, 23, single, 2 children)

Being HIV positive did not mean a woman was always sick, but that she had to work hard for short-term survival. Since many years may pass before full-blown AIDS develops, it is perhaps understandable that HIV could disappear into the background of a woman's life. Although women tried to forget it insofar possible, to the extent that some even said they did not worry and their lives had not been changed, there were still many moments when they could not cope psychologically:

When I've nothing to do, when I'm alone, I just start thinking about it. When there's no one I can talk to, it just comes into my mind. (Judy, 26, boyfriend, 2 children)

Most of the time when I'm at home, and when I wake up during midnight, I start thinking of my kids. (Tendai, 42, divorced, 9 children)

It affects me that most of the people have AIDS. If they die, who is going to live in the world, who will be the mothers and fathers? If we all die, who is going to survive? What will the world look like in the coming years?.... Sometimes when the children are out and me and my husband are discussing about HIV, I feel depressed. (Auxillia, 39, married, 3 children)

What happened to me is that you can think any time you can die. You don't die immediately and you don't live long; it is in between those two things. (Helen, 19, boyfriend, no children)

Most women said their lives (and the lives of their children) had changed drastically because of HIV:

There are so many changes, I cannot think of anything particular. When you know you're HIV positive, you start thinking about your own life. How you value life. Everything is changed, everything. In my brains, I don't know how to explain, but I see that everything is changed. (Judy, 26, boyfriend, 2 children)

I don't know my children will go ahead with school, because I don't know when I will die. (Auxillia)

It messed up my children's future. They were looking forward to be raised by their parents. But now we don't know how it will end. (Chipo, 26, married, 3 children)

It took away my husband and now I am alone with the children. (Barbara, 25, widowed, 3 children)

I could have been bearing a lot of kids. Before I had the virus I never thought about death. (Nyasha, 26, widowed, boyfriend, 2 children)

It changed my whole life. The only period I was happy was when I was married and we had a baby. I have never enjoyed my life. Since I came here my life is terrible. When I came here all my things were stolen. I had plenty of dresses and plenty of shoes. Now I've nothing anymore.... I have nothing to look for, because I know that it becomes worse and I never recover. Why don't I get a chance? I've never been ill and now this is the most terrible disease you can have. (Tsitsi, 31, widowed, one child died)

Emptiness, anxiety and confusion are the prevailing feelings, in addition to the sorrow and anger at the unexpected guest, at themselves, at a husband or boyfriend. Anger and fear may be communicated to one's surroundings, and in any case can cause desolate feelings of doubt, disillusion, and injustice. Women at Sikukuchwa expressed concern for their own well being, about what will happen to them when they have full-blown AIDS, who will care for them and whether they will have to bear a lot of pain. Many families cannot cope with the dying, because they do not have beds and materials:

When I'm at a critical point, who will take care of me? Who will support me with food, work? (Nyasha)

It worries when it takes a long time. When you're ill for a long time, then you better have an accident. To have an accident is better than when you are ill and lie three years in bed. (Chipo)

When you get ill, people will be laughing at you, they don't want to touch you when you mess up yourself, they will be afraid of being with you. There will be no freedom for you. (Sarah, 23, married, 2 children)

I'm afraid to be sick, all those diseases I see people with, especially Herpes Zoster. (Tendai)

I'm always thinking about when will I die. You don't know who will help you when there will be sickness. Relatives will neglect you, so Sikukuchwa will help you. (Tambudzai, 26, single, 1 child died)

I fear there will be no one to love me or talk with me.... that there will be a lack of comfort.... but stigmatization. (women in focus group)

Women knew that when they developed full-blown AIDS, they could receive help from the Sikukuchwa Home Based Care team, which provides care, counselling and material support to anyone with HIV/AIDS. Alternatively, they might find a place in the Care Unit. There a family member could care for them under the supervision of Sr. T., and they would be able to die in at least some dignity, with their family members present. However, women worried more about their children's future than their own – whether their family would be able to care for them, whether they could go to school. Considering the importance of their children to them, their main concerns are not surprising:[2]

There are so many. Where do I get the money for my children to go to school? My sister also has her own kids, so I don't think she can help them financially, because things are already hard with her own kids. (Judy, 26, boyfriend, 2 children)

The first problem for my future is: what about when I'm the first who will develop full-blown AIDS and die, who will look after my kids and give them love as I am trying to do? When it happens, it will be very difficult for them, financially, to have enough food. (Ann)

I don't want to die, because the children are not working. There's no one who can fight for them to survive or get school clothes. That is the biggest problem I'm facing. I'm afraid of dying, because there's no one who can look after my children. I don't have brothers. I have no money for my kids. (Thandi, 41, single, 3 grown-up children)

At the moment I'm a bit worried about myself, because I'm ill sometimes and who is going to care for the kids? I'm praying my mother could have a longer life than me to care for the kids. (Jackie, 31, divorced, 2 children)

Children can make women feel very strong and resolute, wanting to live a long life. They long to see their children growing up and developing, to feel sure they will be able to care for themselves. Yet children were also a major source of stress. Although women were very worried the future of children who were not HIV positive and thus likely to become AIDS-orphans within a few years, only a few had managed to discuss this subject with a close relative; it was still an intention:

I've not spoken with my sister yet about the children. (Chipo)

I've got not yet discussed with her, as time goes on I want to do it. (Jackie)

Helen found herself in a special position. She worried a lot; her boyfriend had asked her to marry him. She was very young (19) and as yet had no children. Having to decide alone about marriage made her feel isolated. She realized the

81

consequences, but also she wanted to lead a normal life, have a husband and bear children – except she did not know if this would be possible.

I think this guy is going to marry me, I'm going to stay with his parents, but my child will be positive. So what am I going to do? So it is difficult. This is the main point that is not making me happy.... I'm afraid, because when I'm HIV positive, does that mean I cannot get any children forever? Because I think if I get married, if I have sexual intercourse, how would he react to me? If I refuse he can beat me. It's difficult to me, so far I'm going to die without child, without any husband. If I'm alone, I sometimes think I'm going to be married now. After that I think it is difficult. He told me: I'm going to marry you. Then I think: I get a positive child. This is causing me big trouble. I said: if you want to marry me, okay, you must marry me, but... (Helen)

Since women generally told no one (or almost no one) they were HIV positive, they had to bear such psychological consequences almost completely alone; this was an additional problem. Almost all indicated that with other sorts of problems, talking to others was their way of coping:

When there's a conflict between me and my husband, I have to find someone to talk to, for relief. Because when I think too much, I get a headache. (Chipo)

Most said they had someone in their social environment with whom they could discuss problems. However, in half of these cases the person did not know they were HIV positive. There were few they could talk to for relief, advice and direct practical help in relation to HIV. Since having HIV without revealing one's seropositive status may lead to feelings of isolation, it is interesting to see in the following chapter how women did manage to cope with HIV and AIDS, even though they scarcely discussed the matter with relatives or friends; this took place almost exclusively with others at Sikukuchwa, who were in the same circumstances.

5 Coping with HIV/AIDS

They went on doing business, arranged for journeys, and formed views. How should they give a thought to anything like a plague, which rules out any future, cancels journeys, silences the exchange of views. They fancied themselves free, and no one will ever be free so long as there are pestilences. (Albert Camus, The plague, 1972)

At present, poor people with HIV cannot hope for a cure; they are progressively forced to come to terms with their illness and symptoms. There are many ways to deal with life's adversities, and most women reported using several coping responses at the same time. This chapter shows women moving from initial coping with HIV to coping with considerable HIV/AIDS in the long term, with considerable differences in coping strategies emerging. The role of social support, including that provided by Sikukuchwa, is then assessed, along with the questions of self help and 'positive living'. The chapter concludes with the women interviewee's comments on what they would like to see happening at Sikukuchwa and for themselves as individuals.

Initial coping responses after the HIV test

Initial reactions to news of being HIV positive were anxiety (9), anger (2), fear (3), confusion (3), denial (2) and sorrow (4). Three women expressed how painful it was:

When the results came out, I thought it was the end of my life. I felt very horrible. (Ann, 23, single, HRD)

I thought: oh God, my husband is HIV positive, my God, we're all going to die. I knew that if he was HIV positive, then I must be positive, too. I started crying and crying. (Nyasha, 26, widowed, HRD)

Tambudzai's reaction was remarkable: she said she was calm and quiet when she heard the news. Probably this had to do with the fact that she was very ill, and did not know the cause. She was delighted that the doctors could say something definitive. Also, she was no longer so worried – after a long period of illness, she had found a place where she felt comfortable. although it was not for long, quite a few women (6) initially thought of suicide:

I was not upset, since I didn't know the disease. I hadn't heard about this, the disease was like an unexpected visitor. So I was quiet to get to know it. I was not afraid, because I was really sick.... Since the doctors told me, I'm not worried anymore. What I'm doing here [at Sikukuchwa] is fine, making jokes and doing some work. (Tambudzai, 26, single, ARC)

I was prepared for the results. I was thinking when they tell me I'm positive I'm going to kill myself. (Judy, 26, boyfriend, PGL)

I thought at first, when I'm positive, I'm going to buy poison. I was upset, but as time goes, I realized that the kids could be lonely and I realized it's only God who is going to keep the children when I die. (Thandi, 41, single, HRD)

I was willing to die before I came to Sikukuchwa, just sitting at home. But at Sikukuchwa I decided that it's not a good way of ending my life. (Christine, 23, divorced, HRD)

Long term coping strategies

Various models have been developed that are relevant to the situation of women who are HIV positive. For example, the complex interplay of biological (reproductive), psychosocial and socioeconomic consequences can be summarized in a 'biopsychosocial' model like that of Wolf et al. (1991). Further, Barnett and Blaikie have described (mainly socioeconomic) ways of coping used by households, families and communities in the face of AIDS. Here the general model developed by Carver et al. (1989) regarding individual's ways of coping with stress will be used as a starting point. Their multidimensional coping inventory, which assesses various ways people respond to stress, is not specific to HIV/AIDS. However, it appears to be suitable for the women interviewed, in particular because of its emphasis on individual coping patterns. The authors use the conceptual analysis of stress and coping offered by Lazarus (1966), who argues that stress consists of three processes. According to Lazarus, *primary* appraisal is the process of perceiving a threat to oneself, *secondary* appraisal is that of calling up a potential response in one's mind, and *coping* is the process of carrying out that response. Lazarus argues that these processes do not occur in strict one two three order; an outcome of one process may re-elicit a preceding process.

Carver et al. (1989) distinguish three general types of coping. *Problem-focused* coping aims at problem solving or otherwise doing something to alter the source of stress. *Emotion-focused* coping is aimed at reducing or managing the emotional distress associated with (or cued by) the situation. Although most stressors invoke both types of coping, problem-focused coping tends to predominate when people feel they can do something about their situation; emotion-focused coping tends to prevail when the stressor is experienced as something that must be endured (Folkman and Lazarus, 1980). Because this distinction proved too simple, Carver et al. have developed 13 conceptually distinct scales. They also separate out functional and potentially less functional properties of coping strategies and add a third type, *'maladaptive'* responses.

This multidimensional coping inventory suggests a way to represent the diverse ways women at Sikukuchwa coped with HIV and AIDS in the long term. As Carver et al. (1989) rightly state, to separate out all of these coping strategies requires having a way to measure and classify them. It was not possible to do this in a formal way; instead I have used the definitions provided by the inventory in a somewhat simplified form. In general, factors other than problem-focused coping can be viewed as variations on emotion-focused coping. The authors emphasize that these factors are often sharply divergent, to the extent of being inversely correlated. For example, denial does not go hand in hand with a positive reinterpretation of events. One main value of the coping inventory is in making such distinctions clear.

The multidimensional coping inventory also has a few weaknesses, which may stem from its American origins. The distinction between problem-focused and emotion-focused coping seems to imply that coping responses are either active or emotional. Yet the authors note that seeking social support for emotional reasons has dual aspects: functional, in offering reassurance, thereby enabling a return to problem-focused coping; and potentially maladaptive – for example, it might be used simply to vent feelings. Emotion-focused coping can also have an active aspect: the women sometimes quite consciously used emotional responses (e.g. positive reinterpretation, acceptance or laughing).

Though Carver et al. present strategies separately, in reality responses overlap; also, people alternate among them. Most women used more than one type of coping at the same time, which might be termed multiple coping responses. Of the problem-focused activities Carver et al. list – active coping (taking direct action), planning, suppressing (screening out) competing activities, restraint coping (forcing oneself to wait before acting) and seeking instrumental social support or assistance – three (active coping, planning and seeking instrumental social support) were used by the interviewees. All five aspects of emotion-focused coping – seeking emotional social support, positive reinterpretation, acceptance, denial and turning to religion – were used. Seeking emotional social support was for the most part directed at other women who participate at Sikukuchwa. Emotional social support is conceptually different from instrumental social support, but in practice, they often occurred together.

The authors' distinction between functional responses and those that tend to be maladaptive is a further limitation of their model, since with HIV/AIDS there are constraints on what one can do to remedy the situation. Therefore I will consider these responses (mental disengagement, behavioural disengagement and focusing on and venting emotions) as simply variations on emotion-focused coping. Often they were in fact valuable, since when used in combination with other coping strategies they enabled additional forms of coping. Moreover, a given coping strategy may well be beneficial for some people in some situations, but not for others. Only one woman turned to behavioural disengagement, but many others sometimes focused on and vented emotions or used mental disengagement to prevent themselves from thinking about HIV/AIDS.

One emotional coping response Carver et al. do not mention, but which was often used by women at Sikukuchwa, was *hope* (for a cure, a longer or better life, or life after death). The only aspect of this desire to put one's trust and belief in something included in the inventory is religion. Yet coping with uncertainty can be aided by hope, belief and trust in any form. Religion is one way to channel these major challenges, and is the entry point offered to HIV-positive women by Sikukuchwa.

The following sections give examples of separate coping responses used by women at Sikukuchwa, while being aware of the existence of multiple coping strategies. Also, HIV/AIDS involves various stages of illness: coping with AIDS is completely different from coping with HIV. The stage (ranging from HIV infection to full-blown AIDS) in which a woman finds herself may influence her search for or need of a particular coping strategy. Therefore in the quotations the women's stage of illness is indicated: asymptomatic (asymp), long-lasting swollen glands (PGL) alone, HIV related diseases (HRD), severe AIDS related complex (ARC) or full-blown AIDS (see Table 2). At the time they were interviewed, most women needed to be coping with HIV, which was generally accompanied by some symptoms. In the list of important characteristics of the women interviewed (Annex 1) the most likely notable response is indicated separately for each woman. In a departure from the list of coping dimensions developed by Carver, I do not distinguish between functional and non-functional coping strategies, and have added the important strategy hope.

Problem-focused coping

People vary in their use of particular coping strategies in particular situations. Being HIV positive is an extreme; no one can fully cope with it. People who want to change their situation often chose problem-focused coping quite consciously, based on a rational decision. However, it is possible only to some extent – actively coping to live a longer life, to make plans and/or seeking instrumental social support to help cope with socioeconomic problems due to HIV. Suppression of competing activities means putting other projects aside and trying to avoid being distracted by other events. This was a limited option for HIV-positive women living in Harare: they had to work hard to make ends meet. Restraint coping in the sense of waiting for an appropriate opportunity to act, holding back and not acting prematurely is also not a sound option in the case of HIV/AIDS. Though Carver et al. consider this an active coping strategy because the person's behaviour is focused on dealing effectively with the stressor, they admit it also has a passive side in the sense that using restraint means not acting. This confirms the interwovenness of problem-focused and emotional coping.

Active coping. This involves active steps to try to remove or circumvent the stressor or alleviate its consequences. HIV-positive women coped actively by caring for themselves to slow the development of full-blown AIDS. This involved caring for your general health, your body, abstaining from sex and changing lifestyles. Because Tambudzai and Noerine used to sell sex, they felt abstention was the most important thing they could do for themselves. Receiving food and money at Sikukuchwa, they were in a position to refuse men. Some others also coped by choosing not to have sex. Perhaps this was a way to feel independent and increase self-respect.

I eat healthy food, every time I check myself when I need more blood, I take juice. When I feel sick, I go straightaway to the clinic. (Christine, 23, divorced, HRD)

I don't care about sex. I've forgotten about that. All I want is to pray. When I walked in the street, a man came to me and said: I love you. I said: I don't want, because you know that there's AIDS. He said: I want to see it, I want to have sex. No, I said, I don't know you, you don't know me. The men don't understand, they say you are a liar. (Noerine, 31, single, HRD)

I don't feel the urge anymore to sleep with many men. The doctors and sisters told me I must use condoms. I've got a box at home, but I'm not using it. I'm just staying like that, I've not any feeling. I haven't got any appetite. When they ask I chase them away. Some follow me. When I become pregnant and they leave me, where can I get money to care for a baby? Social Welfare has no money, so how would I be able to care for a kid? That's why I don't want men. (Tambudzai, 26, single, ARC)

I don't have sexual encounters anymore. I don't go around and am no longer interested. It's not difficult. Whenever you sleep with men, you can wake up in the morning and get ill, pneumonia, sores, wounds. If you go around, you might get STDs on top of the virus. (Joyce, 29, divorced, ARC)

You have to live well, change your lifestyle, change everything. (Chipo, 26, married, HRD)

I don't concentrate on bad things, I take time to rest, I am not thinking about things that can harm my life, I always live positively. (Thandi, 41, single, HRD)

Planning. Planning involves thinking about how to cope with a stressor, coming up with action strategies and thinking about steps to take. The most important thing these women wanted to plan was how to give their children a future. This kept them going, wanting to continue living.

If I found a job, I could work and save money. Because then my child can go to school, because she's the only little one I have left at home. (Tendai, 42, divorced, 9 children, HRD)

I plan a lot for my family, although I don't know what God is going to plan for me. I plan for my kids, I pay funeral order for myself and for my kids, so when one of us dies, the service will help us to bury us. For my baby my aim is, if his health will be good for the coming years, he will go to school, maybe Grade 5, I don't know what God has planned. To go to school and to stay a little bit longer. (Christine, 23, divorced, 2 children, HRD)

My aim is to think, to help myself, not to look for somebody else to look after me. I want to do it myself. If I've got money to buy, to knit, to sell vegetables, buy a machine to sew and you can sell. It's another way of finding money, to help my children. I'm poor, so I can't do it, but I'm thinking of it. (Barbara, 25, widowed, 3 children, HRD)

Yes, I think when I'm here I try to work hard, so that I get experience. When I get experience, I do my own. If I'm serious with dressmaking, it can make me do more in the future. I can do it at home. (Helen, 19, asymp)

Seeking instrumental social support. All women used this type of problem-focused coping – seeking advice, assistance or information from other people – through participation in Sikukuchwa (for examples from Barbara and Marita, see Chapter 4, *Socioeconomic consequences*).

When problems arise I have to talk to somebody who can solve the problem. The more I talk, some will understand my problems and help me in some ways. (Nyasha, 26, widowed/boyfriend, PGL)

Acceptance and ability to control have been said to lead to more active and problem-related coping, whereas emotional coping is thought to occur more often in those who do not accept their illness or do not think it is controllable (Schüssler, 1992). Therefore, it is interesting that, though HIV and AIDS are controllable only to some degree, many women used problem-focused coping.

Emotion-focused coping

Women at Sikukuchwa turned to diverse emotion-focused coping strategies. This section describes the types of emotion-focused coping that Carver et al. consider functional. The next two deal with other variations of emotional coping responses that may be equally adaptive in coping with HIV/AIDS.

Seeking emotional social support. Outside Sikukuchwa most women sought emotional support only in the knowledge they were not the only ones with HIV and from staying with their families. Possibilities for moral support, sympathy or understanding were limited, since outside Sikukuchwa they told few others about their HIV status. For Nyasha, AIDS Awareness programmes were a way of coping; Marita talked only with one HIV-positive woman, at a conference.

- Talking

Talking to others. I'm talking about the virus on and on, just because the more I talk, the more I get used to the virus. I always like talking to people, I don't want to get bored. (Nyasha, 26, PGL)

I have a friend [who is also HIV positive] *with whom I talk about my problems. Sometimes she can help me, sometimes not. So I'm feeling better, because some people live with HIV. (Marita, 22, HRD)*

- Staying with family, especially children. Children are frequently a source of emotional support and closeness for women. Women at Sikukuchwa were very devoted mothers: children were everything to them; they appeared more concerned about their children than about themselves. This was particularly evident in the ways they cared for their children, always wanting be aware of what the child was doing. Perhaps this was why the play garden at Sikukuchwa was right in front of the cooperative. Having children was also very important as a distraction. Women were busy all day reacting to their children, so that they had much less time to think of HIV. In this respect, childcare may be a form of mental disengagement (see below).

Stay with my kids and also with other little children. I tell them stories, laugh and pray. It makes me get better. (Nyasha, 2 children)

Nowadays I'm feeling happy, because my child is walking. She was always sleeping. Nowadays she's running away. And I'm also happy when my husband and I aren't quarrelling. (Sarah, 23, 2 children, ARC)

- Knowing you are not the only one. Many at Sikukuchwa initially thought people in the West could not be HIV positive. After two HIV-positive Canadians visited the support group, they felt even less alone. Some exaggerated the number of HIV-positive people, a phenomenon that has been called *'false consensus'*: people may overestimate the frequency with which their own characteristics, opinions, behaviour or qualities occur (Bosveld et al., 1990). This can be seen as a mild form of denial (see below), which may also serve as a way of coping with HIV/AIDS.

When I went to the conference [for HIV-positive people] *in Mutare, there were many people with HIV. I'm not the only one.... Most of the people are HIV positive. Because there are many people with HIV, I'm not worried. I think a quarter of Zimbabwe is HIV positive. (Marita)*

I always seek for people like me. I'm always searching for my friends (Nyasha, 26, PGL)

I am not alone. There are more. Per day I count more than 30. So almost everyone (Tessa, 23, married, ARC)

I really know it is found in people. I know that each and everyone has got it. I'm not the only one. We are plenty. I'm always listening to radio and TV. And when I'm walking in the roads I see glands and I see he's positive. We are together. We are in the same condition. (Barbara, 25, HRD)

Positive reinterpretation. Positive reinterpretation is aimed at managing the emotions resulting from distress rather than dealing with the stressor. Seeing a stressful transaction in positive terms may subsequently lead to continuation of active, problem-focused coping activities. It can also affect one's conceptualization of the illness and give it new meaning. Two kinds of positive reinterpretation were seen: seeing one's own relatively informed state as an advantage, and seeing positive aspects.

We are better off, because we know we are HIV positive and we are taught about the virus.... When you know it, you can stop with prostitution and care for yourself. Others still walk around. (focus group)

Nobody knows when he dies. An other person can have a car accident tomorrow. (focus group) [Particularly evident at Sikukuchwa, adjacent to the busiest road in Harare, where car accidents happened almost every day!]

I really say it all the time that I have a purpose in life. It's my own choice to tell people about AIDS. If I hadn't HIV, I hadn't the chance to go out and tell people. I know there was a purpose for me of being HIV positive. So I say that's why: God made it for me being HIV positive. I want to put my life in the hands of God. (Ann, 23, HRD, testifying in AIDS Awareness Programmes)

When I was told I was HIV positive, it was a change in my life. For I had been a sinner. Now I want to pray to God and to love him. (Jackie, 31, ARC)

The disease has changed me into a good lady. Before I was full of prestige, always comparing with others. I didn't want to talk to others. Now I try to be good. So the disease might do me something good, you never know. (Nyasha)

It has changed my husband, for he was after sex workers. He went out with other women. Since the diagnosis he doesn't do it. Now he settled down. (Chipo, 26, HRD)

Before the virus I wasn't enjoying sex as since I know it. I enjoy it more than ever.... It's the time to have sex with men. It's sweeter now. (focus group)

Acceptance. Carver et al. (1989) describe this as a response in which a person either accepts the stressor as real (*primary appraisal*) or accepts the absence of active coping strategies (*secondary appraisal*). One might expect acceptance to be particularly important when a stressor is something that cannot be changed. For HIV/AIDS, this is not necessarily negative; it can be seen as a highly adaptive, active coping response that can facilitate active and problem-focused coping. Most women had accepted their HIV status to a large extent and most were fully aware of their responsibilities for themselves and others:

We take it as it is (focus group)

We are staying together with the children, we get food and eat together and we accept that we're HIV positive, not going around to the doctors [i.e. traditional healers]. *(Auxillia, 39, PGL)*

I really worried, but as time went I began to accept it and realize I must live positively. (Nyasha)

Turning to religion. Most Shona people have a rich spiritual world, and many in the group believed in God. The use of religion as a primary coping strategy by so many may also in part have been due to the influence of Sikukuchwa. In any case, an HIV-positive woman may turn to religion and put her trust in God for a variety of reasons. It could serve as a source of emotional support, a vehicle for positive reinterpretation or acceptance, or a tactic for active coping with HIV/AIDS – perhaps looking for a cure or a way to improve one's health. Turning to religion, having faith and devotion to God may be a very adaptive and powerful form of coping, especially when it involves praying with others.

I'm just saying: what is to come is to come. I want to put my life in the hands of God... this disease, it needs praying. We should put our lives in the hands of the Lord. And trust him only. Sometimes I think: this husband ran away and left me with two kids, I have nothing to help myself. Then I just say: it's God's choice to give me that life. It also helps in staying together with others. (Ann)

All I want is to pray only. Because I know there's no other thing I can do. If I say: God, you can help me, I'm sick. You know what to do with me. Then he hears what I'm talking about. When people are talking rubbish to me, I just ignore them. I say: God, you know what you can do with these women, me, I put it in your hands. (Noerine, 31, HRD)

To pray only, when I was thinking I pray to God. When he didn't go to the clinic [her husband did not want to go to collect the results of their HIV tests], *you can pray and you feel better. I pray to God, because he knows it. (Sarah)*

I became a Christian. To pray to God and to love him. I no longer have the appetite to have a man. I'm now trying to be a sister, like Sr. T. [The sisters at Sikukuchwa were a strong example for most women. They symbolized good ways of living and demonstrated living in peace and harmony] *(Jackie)*

The members of the church say: keep on praying to God, it's the only God who makes plans for you. Sometimes it helps me, sometimes not. But when you pray, it will make you free, because you will ascertain that God's spirit is going to come and help you. (Thandi, 41, HRD)

Since my husband died, I started to believe in God and became a Christian. Otherwise you don't survive. There's nobody else for you. I pray very much, in the mornings, in the evenings, to God. That helps me to take the disease as it is.... (Tsitsi, 31, AIDS)

In all cases women felt religion helped. Directly, prayer may stimulate recovery from opportunistic illnesses, forgetting about HIV, coming to terms with the situation and 'taking the situation as it is'. Indirectly, prayer may help people to carry on in difficult periods, and helped some women to stay with others. It was not entirely clear what Christianity implied to them. Most emphasized that their future was up to God, and belief in God sometimes went so far as to support the choice of other coping strategies. Reciprocally, when coping was effective this was seen as the ultimate proof of God's help. Some women handed over all control; for them, these ideas could have increased the risk of fatalism and acted as a barrier to helping themselves. Yet for most women, leaving the future in the hands of God appeared to be a realistic way to accept their condition.

I'm Roman Catholic, they help me. When I am thinking too much about my children and what to give them, I go to the church and talk to God, then I come back feeling well. When I go to church, I can come across people who give me food and pray to God. So God helps me with that. (Barbara)

I go to church once a week, before Sikukuchwa three times a week, also on Thursday afternoon, it's for women only about the husband and the kids. If I pray I feel all right. Religion can help me. If I go to pray, I think less. I think that God is the only person who can help me. If I'm praying there are persons who help me with money. (Tessa, 23 ARC)

Denial. Denial, or refusal to believe the stressor exists (or trying to act as though it is not real) is a somewhat controversial way of coping, which may be beneficial or not. Denial is often seen as useful in the early stages of stressful transactions, but later impedes coping (Levine et al., 1987). Alternatively, in the long term moderate denial (in the sense that only some aspects of the disease are denied, e.g. its potential threat or its uncertainty) may be useful, while either a lack of or an extreme denial may lead to the occurrence of symptoms (Schüssler, 1992). Helen had recently been diagnosed (see also Chapter 2, *Attitudes towards HIV infection....*) – probably the reason for her initial denial. Her parents had passed away and getting money had always been a big problem. Finding money to survive appeared to be more important to her than the problem of HIV/AIDS. Pretty had denied her status for a longer time, probably at least six months (see also Chapter 2, *Attitudes towards HIV infection ....*) She did not often talk about herself, but knew very well what was necessary for an HIV positive woman, as well as her feelings. Her remark below could be seen as typical for someone denying HIV status: it indicates low self-esteem and low self-efficacy to cope more actively with the disease. As a result, denial could become a necessity. When a person is not yet sick, denial may be beneficial. However, when the stressor becomes urgent, denial may create additional problems: it allows the situation to become still more serious, making the coping that eventually must occur more difficult (Matthews et al., 1983).

I do things so I don't lack money. I buy some clothes and sell, so I get money. If I don't buy what I need, I think more. I'm stronger through activities. I feel stronger when I've been working. (Helen, 19, asymp)

The person must know she's not the only one and keep herself healthy. They need care from relatives, because when she's always thinking people run away, she will die of it. And when she can't talk, she will die. (Pretty, 21, asymp)

I don't plan, because otherwise I can slim of it. I'm not going to win, I'm always a loser. When I make plans I can't manage it. (Pretty)

Variations on emotion-focused coping

Although Carver et al. (1989) view a number of coping strategies as less useful (or not useful at all), when it comes to coping with HIV/AIDS I see them as functional: effective and useful in the sense of trying to live positively, or in wishing to live as long as possible with HIV/AIDS (see also *Hope* below). Carver et al. mention that behavioural and mental disengagement presumably function in coping as they do in other domains, such as test anxiety and social anxiety. HIV and AIDS appear similar: insecurity and anxiety are central feelings. Disengagement from a goal may sometimes be a highly adaptive response, particularly when the weak social position of women with HIV taken into account. Women at Sikukuchwa turned to such emotional coping responses in combination with problem- and other kinds of emotion-focused coping.

Mental disengagement. When conditions prevent behavioural disengagement, this variation may occur. A wide variety of activities can serve to distract the person from thinking about the behavioural dimension or goal with which the stressor interferes. Mental disengagement can be seen as a sort of moderate denial (see above); unlike complete denial it can be quite active and conscious.

- Ignoring problems/preventing thinking

Some problems I ignore. Sometimes it succeeds, sometimes it doesn't. (Nyasha, 26, PGL)

I just don't give myself time to think about. (Judy, 26, PGL)

I don't think about being HIV positive. I just take it easy... the more I waste my time on it, the more I get worried and the more I ruin my life. So I always live happy, even with other people who are not positive. (Nyasha, 26, PGL)

When something comes that makes me sad, then I go to a private place and I put it aside, I put it in the hands of God. Sometimes I go to the mirror, see myself and laugh.... Most of the time I want to be happy, free of thinking. Since I'm HIV positive, I don't want to have time to think too much [worry], to have stress. (Ann, 23, HRD)

Tendai is always joking. She cannot be serious. (Judy about Tendai, 42, HRD)

You always see me laughing. I'm always ever happy to forget it myself. Because when I go thinking I'm going to die, it can be rough. I am trying to avoid thinking. When I think too much I will die, that's why you always see me laughing. (Barbara, 25, HRD)

- Avoiding isolation/loneliness

And meet others, so that you aren't isolated and lonely. (Ann, 23, single, HRD)

Some people invite me to their place. (Marita, 22, married, no children, HRD)

And I try not to be alone, because when I'm alone, I start thinking. (Judy, 26, boyfriend, 2 children, PGL)

And when I visit my relatives, I am happy and free. (Tambudzai, 26, single, ARC)

- Escaping through sleep

When I think too much, I want to sleep. I cover my head with the blankets and go to sleep. (Tendai, 41, HRD)

In the evening when I sleep, I can forget. (Tambudzai, 26, ARC)

- Seeking diversion

I have friends [at Sikukuchwa], *we are always laughing, sharing jokes, so that I don't concentrate on the disease. (Chipo, 26, HRD)*

Reading a book before I go to sleep and in the morning. Sometimes at home, I forget I'm HIV positive. When I'm at work, there's nothing. (Judy, 26, PGL)

Especially when I go to the movies, for that time, because that will be the time that I can rest, not thinking of something or what to eat. Then I don't need to think, just because I'm thinking of that cinema. (Pretty, 21, asymp)

For me, it's hard to keep on remembering it. The people I educate through AIDS Awareness want me to lead a normal life, to forget about AIDS. (Ann, 23, testifying in AIDS Awareness Programmes, HRD)

Focusing on and venting emotions. One may focus on distress being experienced and ventilate those feelings: all of the women sometimes turned to crying as a way to cope. Sometimes this led to continued or resumed problem-focused and/or other types of emotion-focused coping. As Carver et al. state, seeking emotional social support is not always useful; focusing on emotions can impede adjustment. However, it may sometimes be functional. A person may use a mourning period to adjust to the loss of a loved one and move on. The emergence of AIDS and subsequent loss of possibilities and capacities could be similar. Tsitsi was not really focused on her emotions, but said she needed to cry:

When I had problems, when I was alone, I closed the doors and the windows and started crying. Now also, that's how I relieve myself from thinking. I cry and I cry, till I have no tears anymore. (Tsitsi, 31, AIDS)

Behavioural disengagement. Behavioural disengagement involves reducing one's efforts to deal with the stressor, even giving up the attempt to attain goals with which the stressor interferes. It is identified with helplessness, and is most likely to occur when people expect poor outcomes from coping. Only Tsitsi, who with full-blown AIDS often felt she did not want to fight anymore, appeared to do this. In addition, Tsitsi's coping behaviour sometimes included focusing on and venting emotions, religion and hope for a cure.

If God would come and we could choose who is going with him and who is going to survive, I would say: take me. This disease is eating you away. I'm only declining and I can do nothing. I'm dying. (Tsitsi, 31, AIDS)

The relationship between behavioural disengagement and development of full-blown AIDS is not clear. In an HIV-positive person negative attitudes, feeling helpless or fully recognizing the course of the disease may affect immuno-logical functioning and cause AIDS to develop more quickly (see next section): developing full-blown AIDS can change a women's attitude into one of giving up.

Hope

Hope is an emotion-focused coping response that is particularly important to those with HIV. Many women coped in part through hoping. Hope often flows from religion or spirituality and may involve having confidence or faith in the future; putting confidence and belief in something unspecified; finding a purpose for living; or trust in, dependence on or devotion to God. Although it may overlap to some degree with other strategies, I consider hope a separate, meaningful category in dealing with HIV/AIDS. It can also be the result of coping: each strategy can result in hope and, consequently, in a positive attitude towards living with HIV. Alternatively, hope may stimulate other coping responses, whether problem-focused or emotional. Coping with anxiety and uncertainty can be aided by hope, belief and trust. Religion is a way to channel these big challenges, and is precisely the entry point offered by Sikukuchwa.

Hope can help people survive, as an AIDS support organization in Uganda also stresses: 'Hope lifts your spirits and gives you strength to face each situation. Hope can help you fight HIV and AIDS and live longer' (TASO et al., 1991). Being HIV positive changed the purpose in life of the women interviewees, gave them a purpose or made it more pronounced. Many said they lived more consciously and also more day by day, not knowing how many days were left. Janifa is an example of a woman choosing her own way of life. This seems appropriate as long as she makes the choice herself, respects decisions made by other women and takes responsibility for others – all aspects emphasized at Sikukuchwa.

It causes me to do everything, because when I'm dead, I can't do it anymore. You must do it when you're still alive. (Judy)

I can't prevent getting infected with HIV anymore. Me and my husband are going to enjoy it to the last and decided not to use condoms. We are already dead. (Janifa, not included in the sample)

- Hope for a cure (see also Tsitsi, Auxillia and Chipo in *Attitudes towards HIV infection….*, Chapter 2), or to live longer in general

I always wait for the answer of the Lord. He might let the scientists find a cure for the illness. Or he just says: you'll die. So then I die. So I'm patient. I might die or the cure may be found. (Nyasha, 26, PGL)

I am praying to God to keep me, so the kids will be old and seeing me as a grandmother. My aim is to work for the kids. I hope they will be old enough to look after themselves when I die. (Thandi, 41, single, 3 children, HRD)

My purpose is to keep on going to the church, so that God adds some of my days, so I can keep my kid and live strong. (Joyce, 29, divorced, ARC)

It's not the end of the world, of your life. There are so many days left and everyone dies. It's not for you to think about it, it's only God who knows when your time arrives. It's God's duty. He's the one who gave me life. It's just like when you plant flowers. When you want to put them in the vase, you're the one who chooses the flower you want. That's how it is with life. So he decides when he takes it back. (Judy, 26, PGL)

My will is that God lets me live a bit longer, so that I can care for my kids. For my mother is staying in the rural areas with the kids, but I support them to enlighten the burden of my mother. I can't support them here [in town], because it's too expensive. (Jackie, 31, divorced, 2 children, ARC)

- Hope for a better life

I want to have a long life and a new life. (Sarah, 23, ARC)

To have a better life, I need a big room and the room furnished. I need the property to go back and forget about the disease. I need to work hard, to do something. (Nyasha, 26, PGL)

- Hope for life after death

This is not our permanent life. Because when I think of life, we are just waiting, like a bus stop, just waiting for the bus to pick us up. When I think about death, I'm going to start a new life, which is better. (Judy, 26, PGL)

Coping in stages

Coping strategies vary over the course of the illness: a woman must change her responses when circumstances change and a particular strategy is no longer sufficient. For example, when she becomes quite sick, denial is not possible. Coping develops in stages, which might be termed *incremental coping*. To illustrate this process I would like to focus on Tsitsi's story. She had once worked among the others in the cooperative, a beautiful and intelligent woman who seemed to think often about the course of her illness. When Mary, another participant, had full-blown AIDS and was admitted to the Care Unit, her relatives did not want to take care of her. Tsitsi took over this task and started to live with Mary in the ward (see also Chapter 3, *Absolute secrecy*):

Sr. T. asked others, but they didn't want to. I realized that next time it [full-blown AIDS] could happen to me. Today it's me, tomorrow you. (Tsitsi, 31, AIDS)

Mary sometimes acted obstinate and unstable, which was probably related to AIDS:

Maybe it's the disease in her head, I don't know. (Tsitsi)

Tsitsi's knowledge of full-blown AIDS came from this experience. Soon she was a patient in the Care Unit herself. Although she tried to find a way to cope, a new balance, this was nearly impossible. Her dominant thought was that nothing could be done for her. In June 1993 her mother came to the Care Unit and cared for her for a few months. When her mother went back to the rural area, Tsitsi became terminally ill and died before her mother could return. Tsitsi died February 1994, after a long and lonely period of illness.

I think too much. How can I not think when I know I'm dying? I'm thinking of my mother, who had a terrible life, she's always worrying about me, she has no job, she's divorced. Of my brothers, of myself, I never felt happy. You know, when they knew I had the disease, they chased me. I think very much. How can I accept it and not think when I continuously feel the pain?.... I know I shouldn't think too much, because that progresses the disease. So I have to find some diversion. I used to have my husband to talk with, but now he's dead. (Tsitsi)

This is the illness, nothing recovers anymore. Actually I should have an operation for my piles, but that can cause me to die. (Tsitsi, 18-05-'93) I have no hope to recover, I only know I'm dying. (02-06-'93) I don't want to wait. I feel already dead. I have nothing to look for, because I know it becomes worse and I never recover. I only want to see my mother, then I can die. (Tsitsi, 02-06-'93)

When a woman is admitted in the Care Unit as an AIDS patient, a new way of coping is required. But finding a new balance is very difficult when you are always sick and must live with ups and downs. These differ greatly among individuals; illnesses can change every day. This, as well as the continuing pain and knowledge that the disease cannot be cured, is very difficult. Coping with HIV/AIDS should be seen as a dynamic process, its nature shifting from stage to stage as the disease progresses: from news of being HIV positive, via the asymptomatic stage, persistent generalized lymphadenopathy, HIV related diseases, and severe AIDS Related Complex to the terminal stage of HIV infection – the development of full-blown AIDS (see also Table 3).

After settling in at Sikukuchwa most women seemed to accept their condition (HIV positive without too many symptoms) and were able to cope with their infection quite well. Being HIV positive one needs to look after oneself carefully, as well as the children; to go to hospital or clinic; and to feel responsible for others. But all had moments when it was impossible to cope, in particular when something serious happened either to themselves, their children, another woman or child at Sikukuchwa, or a relative. There was always the threat that they could have full-blown AIDS the next day. When they were ill, this seemed especially real. This was why even when they said they were coping some women were worried at the same time:

I'm afraid of the disease, sometimes. Sometimes, I think too much, when I see sick people. (Judy, 26, PGL)

When I get sick, I get worried. I always think: oh, I might be going in the wrong direction, I go on the wrong road. I don't know when things come. When my child is ill, then I think: oh, maybe it has come to the point. (Nyasha, 26, PGL)

I'm not feeling well, I think about HIV, my husband is ill. I think, I don't want to explain... (Sarah, 23, ARC)

Even if a woman is coping with HIV at a particular moment, it is not certain she will accept the next phase to the same extent. For most women, although they were continuously confronted with women with full-blown AIDS in the Care Unit, it was still impossible to be fully aware of the consequences of their situation. Many closed their eyes to the symptoms and emotions of these women, so interactions with them remained superficial. This was not necessarily a wrong or less useful coping response. On the contrary, it might be a functional, a kind of natural protective mechanism. If an HIV-positive person fully realizes the expected course of her disease, life is harsh and it may speed the development of full-blown AIDS.

Looking at coping with HIV/AIDS as an incremental process suggests that even when women who appeared to be at similar points in the development of HIV/AIDS may not have been in comparable coping stages. This makes it very difficult to assess coping responses. Moreover, Carver et al. (1987) have suggested the importance of individual differences in coping. For example, it is not known whether or to what extent personality characteristics play a role in the choice of a given strategy. Nor is it clear whether there is a systematic relationship between personality and the patterns, sequences and changes in coping over time (Carver et al., 1987).

Coping, personality characteristics and support

Social and psychosocial support, information and counselling benefit coping. Women who were counselled intensively at the moment of HIV diagnosis appeared to have coped better with their HIV infection than those with little or no counselling. They more often told others about their HIV infection and used a greater variety of coping strategies than women who were not counselled. They more often used problem-focused coping, in particular seeking instrumental support, combined with emotion-focused coping, such as acceptance, seeking emotional support and positive reinterpretation, but also mental disengagement. All turned to religion and hope as ways of coping.

Coping may in turn favour the presence and use of social support. Apart from influencing the course of the disease (Schüssler, 1992) and one's emotional state, coping can influence the perception of social support (Wolf et al., 1991), and ability to cope effectively may increase the availability and quality of such support (Wortman, 1984). The construction and use of a social network can thus be seen as an expression of the woman's control, self-efficacy and social competence (Schüssler, 1992), reflecting her personal coping style. Self-efficacy, social competence and emotional stability are generally associated with problem-focused coping, and social withdrawal with negative emotional coping (Schüssler, 1992). Although most women did not communicate their HIV status to their community, and most used emotional coping, it would be wrong to conclude that this was negative emotional coping. On the contrary, useful emotional coping as defined by Carver et al. (1989), supplemented by a number of other functional emotion-focused coping strategies, was most often seen. Although their self-efficacy and social competence towards their social environment was low, during the research period all appeared to cope quite well with their illness. Even those who had not been counselled seemed to have found useful ways of coping through the interaction and support received at Sikukuchwa.

The role of support provided by Sikukuchwa

At Sikukuchwa people can protect themselves to save their lives. They save their lives through being here. (Noerine, 31, single, former sex worker)

Sikukuchwa means the starting of a new life. You leave everything before you were knowing that you are HIV positive and you start to think and act positively. (Judy, 26, 2 children, boyfriend)

In addition to learning about HIV-positive women, their coping strategies and their needs for support, objectives of this study were to gather information about the amount and quality of support provided by the Sikukuchwa project and to propose supplementary measures for possible improvements in support, as well as giving an assessment that might be useful for similar projects.

To meet needs for support, Sikukuchwa set up counselling, income-generating activities (for women only), care, and the support (self help) group discussed in a later section. The project thus not only assisted women with economic (financial, instrumental and material support) and social (education and information, initiation of a support group, company) support, but also with psychological support (warmth, affection, love, encouragement, emotional support). This can be particularly important, since as noted earlier psychosocial stress can have immunosuppressive effects. Social support and self-help groups can directly affect immunological function or serve as a buffer against stress by enhancing coping effectiveness, self-esteem, motivation and/or engagement in health-promoting behaviour (Lazarus and Folkman, 1984; Stewart, 1990).

Initial support

As described in Chapter 2, almost all came to Sikukuchwa because someone told them about the project or invited them to come. If they did not, some women were visited again by Sikukuchwa's Home Based Care team. No one was seeking emotional support or intended to find a self-help group. Instead, most said they had been just staying at home, felt isolated and were afraid to talk to anyone about their disease. When they heard about Sikukuchwa, most came immediately, but some waited for months before daring to come. The first day was often one of relief and disbelief.

In April '92 the doctor tested me and told me about Sikukuchwa. Only in September I went, because I was shy. Every Thursday the HBC team visited me, from April to September. I was shy, I did not really wanted to come to Sikukuchwa. Now not anymore, I get up with others. I was shy, because at that time I thought there was only a small number of people with HIV, I didn't know that everyone could get affected. I was thinking I was the only one. (Tessa, 23, married)

The sisters received me as if we had met already, if they knew me long ago, not as a stranger. It helped me, because when I came here I was helpless, didn't know what to do. But when Sr. T. counselled me, I accepted the situation. That was a relief, that's when I started to learn to live with it.... At the cooperative, they received me warmly, everyone was trying to help me and encouraged me to come every day. When I first saw them, they were laughing and nobody seemed to worry. When Sr. T. said they were HIV positive, I thought she wanted to cheer me up. I didn't believe it: how can they laugh when they are positive? (Judy, 26, boyfriend)

Almost all women knew others who were HIV positive but did not want to come to Sikukuchwa. The focus (discussion) group suggested reasons:

Some are shy, or in denial - some just ignore it, some haven't heard about Sikukuchwa, men do not allow, they don't want to be known, they are afraid of telling anybody or they are afraid of facing reality. (focus group)

Sometimes they don't know about Sikukuchwa. Others are workers, so they don't have the time. But I know many of them are shy, because at the clinic they tell about Sikukuchwa, how they help, but many of them don't like to come here. Because Sikukuchwa is a place where everybody knows it's for HIV-positive people, because it's published at the radio and TV. So when you say, others will know. People talk about Sikukuchwa, they see radio and TV, for example they saw Ann. They think there will be a time they have to talk in the videos. (Tessa)

Initially, most women came mainly in search of instrumental social support. One aim of Sikukuchwa Care Trust is to provide basic medication and a feeding scheme for women and their children. A holistic approach is used, on the assumption that HIV-positive women cannot live positively with HIV/AIDS, trying actively to cope, unless their basic needs have been satisfied. This is also emphasized by Sr. T.

In the rural area they grow crops and have free accommodation. We don't have food in town, so we are lucky to have Sikukuchwa. (Auxillia, 39, married, e.c. 5)

Before I came here I was thin, but Sikukuchwa has made me strong. Now I'm not always sick. (Tendai, 42, divorced, e.c. 1)

To help me. What you want, you can get. Because my husband has no job, I need something which helps me, porridge with peanut butter, beans. If I hadn't come here, my baby would have died. I earn some money by sewing and knitting and they give me food. At home I didn't knit and sew. This time I do it all together. (Sarah, 23, married, e.c. 3)

When I'm suffering I go to Sr. T. Then she gives medicines. Here at Sikukuchwa you can see the doctor every week. If you stay at home, you can't see a doctor, then you have to pay money. I didn't have the money to pay for those schools where you can learn dressmaking. But here I get experience and secondly, if we have money we share it. I want to do something which can help me. If you have money to start, you can do things on your own. (Helen, 19, boyfriend, e.c. 3)

Sikukuchwa uses a holistic approach. We believe you cannot give advice when people have nothing to eat. Therefore most times I give something when I counsel a person. People cannot care if they do not have anything. (Sr. T., one of Sikukuchwa's two coordinators)

Although the aim is to provide assistance for women who have lost the support of relatives and neighbours because they are HIV positive, Sr. P. of the Home Based Care team said that in practice referral is not generally limited: almost all women attending a clinic or a hospital in a high-density area have little assistance or support, whether HIV positive or not. Poorer women are more willing to come to Sikukuchwa, perhaps due to their greater need for material support, but better-off women may need emotional support.

Support needed and received

In addition to instrumental social support, other types of support offered by Sikukuchwa may be even more important to the women. The focus group summed up support through care, comfort, counselling, communication and education (support group and prayer group, see also Introduction, *Dawn of a new life*), food, and from creating an income, e.g. sewing and knitting in the cooperative (see also Introduction, Dawn of a new life). Ann even said HIV influenced her life positively, but only because she came to Sikukuchwa. Such coping is referred to above as positive reinterpretation.

When I came to Sikukuchwa, Sr. T. gave me a blood test. After two weeks the results came back and I was HIV positive. She said: when you have HIV, you must accept it. Love your husband. For I've been blaming my husband that he brought the disease. (Nyasha, 26, widowed/boyfriend, 2 children, e.c. 4, PGL)

The sisters give love and say don't think of many things. And support yourself, let's say when you are worried. They make you feel well, refresh your mind. We discuss HIV, there are many others. It helps me. At home I was just sitting and caring for the kids. I had no way of getting money and other things. At the cooperative I saw people just like me and we share ideas and refresh our minds. (Tessa, 23, married, 2 children, e.c. 5, ARC)

Life has changed, because when I was at home, I didn't have anything to eat. I was always sick and asleep and thus had no time to look for money. But since I'm here I'm strong, finding things to sell, from that money I can support my kids. (Thandi, 41, single, 3 children, e.c. 1, HRD)

The others in the cooperative welcomed me, saying: here you will be okay. This is a place where you can forget some of your problems. It was helpful for me to learn about how to sew and to knit and I could forget all my problems. I got money for rent each month. (Tsitsi, 31, widowed, no children, e.c. 2, AIDS)

If it haven't been for my HIV positivity, I wouldn't have come to Sikukuchwa. I would be struggling, I said I had a very difficult life, it wasn't enough to sell vegetables and tomatoes. So with Sikukuchwa I had a new chance in life. The time I was positive, it was a chance of getting enough. Where can I get cooking oil, food for the children. When I started to participate in the project, I didn't feel alone anymore: here there were women with whom I could share my illness. I used to think I was the only one... now I can talk about it with other women, who are different, but share the disease. If I wasn't positive, most of the people wouldn't know me [through AIDS Awareness Programmes]. So some people know me through AIDS, they are friends through AIDS. The time I came here, I often thank God for that. (Ann, 23, single, 2 children, e.c. 4, HRD)

The cooperative works like a self-help group: sharing in income-generating and other activities, women meet others in similar situations. Most stay a long time, because the emphasis is not on a job or on money but on emotional support, which Sikukuchwa's management considers at least as important as earnings. When you see women from their arrival until a few months later, the impact of the programme is clear. Women relax and become less frightened, opening up and sharing experiences. They really do have a new life, basically because Sikukuchwa gives them a chance. It was noteworthy (but logical) that women who did not communicate with anyone except others at Sikukuchwa about being HIV positive leaned most heavily on the material and emotional support of the project:

Since I've been diagnosed HIV positive, the sisters gave me accommodation. When I've got problems, I go to Sr. T., she's my mother and father.... I don't foresee any problems, because I've got the sisters [of Sikukuchwa] near, they will help my child. (Joyce, 29, divorced, 1 child, e.c. 1, ARC)

If something has upset me, I always go to Sr. T. and tell her my problems, since I've nobody at home. She tells me if you keep on thinking you get sick. It enlightens my heart to tell someone. If you tell, it will come out of your mind, but otherwise you keep on worrying. (Judy, 26, boyfriend, 2 children, e.c. 4, PGL)

The most important thing Sikukuchwa does is that it's a cooperative and a support group. And when I have got problems, I can go to our sisters. (Noerine, 31, single, no children, e.c. 1, HRD)

I'm happy that Sikukuchwa can keep me, because when I was at home, who is going to keep me? I got money to buy the rent, for food and even to go to the clinic, you need money. And when you are sick, like me, you need tablets. Where could I buy them? They give me food, accommodation, treat me, I'm thankful for that. (Tsitsi)

Sikukuchwa tried to stimulate women to do things themselves; for example, a plot to grow vegetables to used at home or sell. Second-hand clothes could also be kept or sold. Once a week Sikukuchwa organized prayer group meetings, presided over by two novices. Management put a lot of emphasis on coping through prayer, but left the choice to the women. Sr. T. said most women at Sikukuchwa were very religious and glad when someone prayed with them, and women said prayer meetings certainly helped.

The women are very keen on God. They could be angry, but they are not. They have accepted their condition to a large extent. What else do we have to offer? (Sr. T., one of two Sikukuchwa coordinators)

Because I want to learn more about the word of God. When you are praying, you can feel the presence... You won't be afraid of anything. You just say: God, I put everything in your hands. You can do what you want with my life. (Judy)

They help me to pray to God, to lead a new life. God is my help, he can know what I think. When something bad is happening, you pray. Then my heart will be open. (Sarah, 23, married, 2 children, e.c. 3, ARC)

Sometimes I think too much and when I come to pray I think less, because I know Jesus is the one who can help me. He's the one who can really satisfy my needs. Sometimes I'm ill and when I pray I feel better, because I believe in that God. They teach us many phrases from the Bible, sometimes love. Sometimes I hate other people, at home or here at the cooperative. When they read I think I'm doing wrong to somebody. When you love other people, you love yourself, that's what I like most. (Tessa)

There was a great deal of interaction at Sikukuchwa. Women saw each other almost every day, making comparisons among themselves and some gossiping inevitable. This seemed quite frequent and had become quite a problem for the coordinators. Therefore it was not surprising that my questions about things the women did not like produced the following references to negative social exchanges. Nevertheless, the support group and other activities had a strong therapeutic effect.

Africa differs from Europe in that in Africa they're very jealous. They are very jealous. When everything was stolen and I got a dress from Sikukuchwa, they were very jealous. But of what? I had nothing. When I got shelter they talked. Everyone is always talking. But they don't say it directly, they are only gossiping with others. And then the other comes to me saying: Tsitsi, do you know that... said... about you? Who?... And then I was surprised. And when I ask they just say no. (Tsitsi)

If you say something at Sikukuchwa, it is spread. About clothes, how you look like and other things. In our culture, they are jealous. About everything, they start at school. When you are not there, they are gossiping. (Tessa)

I'm especially disappointed when people don't do things they really want, when they talk about someone who is not around, when they upset me. I don't like people who talk about someone who is not around. (Pretty, 21, divorced/boyfriend, 1 child, e.c. 3, asymp)

When I stay here, others can talk to you rubbish questions, others they can shout at you. (Noerine)

The support group

The 'support group' was established by the sisters of Sikukuchwa as a means of self help. It consisted of an HIV-positive chairperson, secretary and treasurer/vice-chair and some 30 other HIV-positive participants in the cooperative. The support group met each week for two hours with the chairperson presiding. It helped in much the same way as the cooperative, but was only for HIV-positive women. Staying together, talking and venting emotions all helped. Further, it provided a more structured way for women to educate themselves, share ideas and communicate. In 1993 it was still new, but had already proved its value. Members were encouraged to deal openly with their status. For example, in one focus group discussion (08-07-1993), everyone introduced themselves as 'Dinonzi... (My name is....) and I am HIV positive'. Only Pretty did not attend the support group. She said it was only for HIV-positive people. Helen did not attend often; Nyasha said she was not really interested because she was still too young. In the focus group others agreed the group helped them very much.

To get help for myself. I got the support of being told how to live positively and why I should live positively. We are with more and can share things. They advised me how I should help myself, how I can stay, not drinking beer, not smoking cigarettes, not to go to those doctors who stay in homes, those back door doctors [traditional healers and herbalists]. (Tsitsi, 31, widowed)

In the support group we learn more than with counselling. From discussing with others, you learn more. The support group is the main thing which helps me. Sometimes we take books and learn about STD, how we can help ourselves. In the support group you have the knowledge and you can read from books. I'm not educated and cannot read books, so I have to talk and listen to know. Because we go to the support group with HIV positives only, we can talk about the matters and share ideas about how to care safe and food to eat. And we talk about the numbers of people with HIV, especially here. (Tessa, 23, married)

It can help me, because it's where I can get experience about people with HIV, about the symptoms you get. And what you should do when you have HIV. They talk about if you're HIV positive, you must eat vegetables, matemba [dried fish]. If you've got a partner, you can use condoms. I'm participating in the support group to know how I can react in my life, if I'm HIV positive, to give advice to other people, to share ideas. Don't do sexual intercourse with many people. (Helen, 19, boyfriend, in an individual interview)

To learn something, to talk, to pray and do something. Nowadays I want to establish a garden of vegetables for the support group. When we have enough money, we share it for the support group. From the money we buy something from the cooperative and sell it again. When someone dies you can take money to go to the funeral and take millet meal and vegetables for them. When some- one is in hospital, we go and buy bananas, oranges and everything to give her. On Wednesday we collect Z$ 1 or 50 cents for the support group. When my baby was in hospital they also came. (Sarah, 23, married)

Nevertheless, the group faced many difficulties. Since the onset, members had sought a useful structure. Things were always happening (a burial, absence of the chair or vice-chair, an important visitor, work that had to be finished), so it was difficult to fix a meeting day. It also took time before the meetings became structured and provided specific support. Presiding over a large group calls for experience that none of the women had; sometimes everyone talked at once and people did not really listen to each other. Some talked all the time and others did not dare say anything. Often many subjects were discussed at the same time, making in-depth discussion difficult. It was not clear how many members were satisfied. Soon the group was deliberating its goals and priorities and experimenting with more adequate ways to hold meetings.

Self-help aspects

Women found the self-help aspect one of the most important features of Sikukuchwa. The focus group said they felt stronger due to organizing them- selves, because they have the same problem. Some also felt stronger because they believed they could do something about their situation. As Stewart (1990) notes, self-help groups can alleviate feelings of *stigma*, provide a *supportive community* for sharing a stigmatized attribute and counteract feelings of *lone- liness* by offering compensatory social ties:

It's just by knowing I'm not alone, so I must not worry about it. I thought I was the only one. By knowing other people are also HIV positive, I feel stronger. But that doesn't mean I'm happy that other people are also HIV positive. (Judy) Every week there's a new person at Sikukuchwa, so we can see we are with many. Because in my mind I was thinking there are so few and I'm dying. Now I see many, almost the whole world. Now I don't mind, because it's spreading into the whole world. (Tessa)

When you meet other people who have the same disease as you, you can relax. That's the cure. (Nyasha)

Individuals seek out others who share the same experience to help define and comprehend their reactions. Self-help groups meet needs for *affiliation* and offer opportunities to *express feelings*.

At home there was no one to share. It enlightened my heart when I came to Sikukuchwa. (Ann)

Because we know the woman with whom we talk has got the virus, too. So we get strong, to talk with each other. (Noerine)

Normally, you hear another idea of someone, instead of sitting alone. Because whenever you are alone, you have to think of someone, your child or your husband [who had died]. *When you stay together, the days are going on. (Tsitsi)*

If I'm here, I don't think too much. It can help me, because when we are talking I'm feeling well. Because we're the same. At home there's no one to tell the problem, because it's a secret. Here everybody knows, so I'm free to talk. It can help me by talking with others, sharing ideas, seeing other people, just see them. (Tessa)

I'm happy when I'm here, because we share each others' mind about the problems. (Thandi)

When I'm here, I feel that I'm with my ladies and I can say everything I want. When I have problems, I tell my friends at Sikukuchwa, so they give a hand with the problems. (Christine)

Obtaining help by joining with others who have similar problems creates a sense of control over one's life and movement towards advocacy, a sense of *empowerment*. Empowerment also includes a feeling of insight and understanding:

They help me to forget about that virus.... Because it helps me to know about my life and to learn about myself: how to make healthy, how to protect yourself, to cook smart things, to clean your body, to ignore sex, to clean our houses, to wash my toilet, to sweep my room, to wear clean clothes, to make our beds neat. You know when you have a virus, you must not have sex with men, eat proper food, wash your body. And when somebody says you've got HIV, you should ignore him. And when you have a boyfriend and you don't know if he's all right, you must use condoms and protect yourself from STDs. (Noerine)
When I get home, I think about it, but if I'm here I don't think too much. And we're talking about it. It helps, because we're the same. Sometimes you understand it and get the meaning of being HIV positive, you discuss it with others at Sikukuchwa. But if you don't get the sense, you continue thinking about it. (Tessa)

Significant relationships created through self-help groups promote *positive reflected appraisals* and enhance *self-esteem*:

I have friends, we're always laughing, sharing jokes, so that I don't concentrate on the disease. (Chipo)

For we have the same in common, it's good. We know each other. We feel stronger together, because our problems are the same. And by seeing so many. (support group, 08-07-'93)

Through Sikukuchwa I learned to be patient. Through Sikukuchwa I got friends. (Nyasha)

Since I'm HIV positive in 1989, I've been in Nyanga and I had no friends to talk to about my problems. But then I came here, I got a friend who is HIV positive. (Marita)

These sentences reflect the emotional coping response of positive reinterpretation: seeking others in the same situation, redefining the disease to see positive aspects and seeing that you are not alone. Self-help group members increase their well being by making *downward comparisons* with the less fortunate to enhance self-esteem and *upward comparisons* with effective coping models in the reference group:

Because we share problems, because we have the same problem. When someone has a problem, you can see how she solves it, you can see how other people do. And when you think you have problems and you see others, then my problems are better. Because it relieves my mind, when I'm worried it helps, it becomes less. (Judy)

In a way, the support group satisfied some criteria of a *social movement*: opposition from society (real or perceived, discussed in Chapter 3), a sense of common purpose, need for both individual and social change, and empowerment (Stewart, 1990). However, empowerment and need for social change did not lead women to 'come out' in their communities and educate others, although many considered this a common purpose (see below).

Positive living

Sikukuchwa's work focuses on the concept of 'positive living': taking care of body, mind and soul to secure a healthier, happier and more fulfilling life. The first public health messages in Zimbabwe (Beware of AIDS, AIDS kills) negatively affected attitudes towards those with HIV/AIDS. There were no messages about those with HIV. Positive living was Sikukuchwa's way of emphasizing living rather than dying with AIDS, and quality of life rather than quantity. This philosophy had been stated earlier by TASO, in Uganda (TASO, 1991): people can live positively by making healthy choices, making the best of life, living as normally as possible and looking after spiritual and mental health. Because it has to do with attitudes rather than knowledge, living positively is difficult to describe. Each woman had her own explanatory model:

Just leave everything you have been doing. Let's say if you have been drinking, many boy friends, smoking, just leave them. And don't give yourself time to think too much. And also don't think about tomorrow and leave it for that day and live it for the full. Not thinking what will I eat or wear. Just leave it for tomorrow and see when it comes. (Judy)

Positive is when you have the symptoms of the virus, you have to accept it, the symptoms, the pain, the diarrhoea. (Noerine)

At the time I was told, I couldn't really believe it. I was thinking sometimes the doctor made a mistake. So I came to believe I'm positive, meaning: I really believe I've got HIV and I really accept it. The starting of a new life. (Ann)

Not to go around with men, to be smart, washing hands, eating fruits, keeping clean, not compete with those who are not HIV positive, eat well and not think too much. (Joyce)

What is happening here is that people are suffering, but when time goes, the person feels better. When she comes here, you think that the person is going to die. (Helen)

You can live positively by eating balanced food, vegetables, white meat, not red, matemba, so you don't get full-blown AIDS quickly, but live for some time. (Tsitsi)

Accept it. Live with it and do not spread it. (focus group)

In Western society, positive living means new cognitive goals, enrichment of life, doing 'good', mobilization of self-help groups, coming out together, fighting, actively working for prevention, travelling. Western values and norms suggest these are all important – and in the West they are affordable. But positive living also means living 'for the day' – something closer to the meaning for women at Sikukuchwa. They found happiness in basic things such as having enough food and money and being able to care for their children. Probably this was why most felt they were already living positively.

I don't know if I'm living positively. I'm just living as I was before, the only difference is that I come to Sikukuchwa. I was not drinking beer, not having many boyfriends, so I don't know how I can change. It was just the same as before: think of today, don't worry about tomorrow. (Judy)
I think positive living means positively as we are. So you must live positively. Now I know I'm positive, so I'm caring for myself, eating good food and not thinking too much. I learned to live positively, because I don't think too much about HIV. (Tessa)

But compared to the West, how can we live positively if we are poor? (Ann)

Common purposes for the future

Sikukuchwa was expanding, and a new building offered housing for more AIDS patients, a larger room for the children's playgroup and private rooms for women workers in the cooperative. Women suggested only a few additional things they would like Sikukuchwa to do in the near future, primarily taking care of them when they have full-blown AIDS and looking after their children or providing shelter for them (see Chapter 4, *Psychological consequences*):

The children will suffer when I'm not there. If Sikukuchwa was able to take care of them when I'm dead. (Tendai)

Nothing, but I can say I want Sikukuchwa to continue and the cooperative to grow and I want the sisters to stay. They give us time to refresh our minds here at Sikukuchwa. (Tessa)

Continue helping and loving us. (focus group)

As HIV-positive people, the women also thought they could do something themselves by making others aware of HIV/AIDS and encouraging people with HIV to get support and live positively. To this purpose, Ann, Nyasha and Marita were testifying in AIDS awareness programmes and attended a conference for HIV-positive people. Ann also sent a proposal for a poster at a symposium in France. I was able to translate the reply she received – there was no money for her travel. Other potential funders she approached also could not help. As an HIV-positive woman, Ann had something to contribute, but her initiative failed. Others did not speak out in their wider environment. Jackie indicated she would like to educate people, but only those who did not know her. She, like others, was afraid of being recognized by people in her own area who might discriminate:

I want to educate the people. But where can I go to explain? Then I have to go to places where people don't know me, like Masvingo. But not in this area, I'm too popular, I have stayed and worked in Harare for a long time. (Jackie)

I may educate people, but not saying I've got the virus. I want to educate that they should protect themselves. (Chipo)

You just tell others AIDS is there and that they must value their life: it's special. And to tell others who are HIV positive that they must not worry. (Judy)

I'm encouraging people to live positively. (Joyce)

Although women such as Jackie, Chipo and Joyce (and Judy, who had started to give testimony in AIDS Awareness programmes but still did not talk to people in her direct environment), said they wanted to help others with HIV and to educate the general public, they did not do so in practice. Here there was still a mission to fulfil: one thing Sikukuchwa might do is to encourage such women to talk privately with others who are HIV positive but not yet included in the project.

6 Major findings and discussion

Staying at Sikukuchwa and talking with the HIV-positive women there created a unique possibility to experience their process of coping with HIV and AIDS from close by. The individual stories of 19 women living with HIV/AIDS made clear how difficult it is to generalize on the consequences of and ways of coping with HIV infection. Nevertheless, some conclusions can be drawn. A careful reading of Appendix 1 plus the women's own words in the quotations throughout the Bulletin (page numbers are listed in the last column of the Annex) allow a more nuanced view of the overall results and conclusions than can be presented in this chapter. The women, who were themselves receiving psychological, social and economic support, thus provide rich material for others to learn from their circumstances and experiences.

Coping with their illness appeared a complex task for women with HIV/AIDS at the Sikukuchwa project. They used a combination of emotion-focused and problem-focused coping, sometimes using several strategies at once and some-times shifting among strategies over time. Problem-focused coping responses included active coping and planning for the future of one's children; most often, however, women used emotion-focused coping (religion, positive reinter-pretation, acceptance, seeking of emotional social support, and denial). Accep-tance of one's own illness appeared to be something completely different from willingness to reveal an HIV status to relatives, friends and others in their com-munity: women did this hesitantly or not at all. Moreover, emotional social sup-port was largely sought from other women at Sikukuchwa. Turning to religion was a common coping style, which may have been influenced by Sikukuchwa. Two extreme variants of emotion-focused coping strategies, used in alternation by many women, were mental disengagement and hope. The division proposed by Carver et al. (1989) therefore seems somewhat forced: the fact that women used several coping strategies at once and switched among styles demonstrates how difficult it is to separate problem-focused and emotion-focused coping responses. Nor did a distinction between useful and less useful coping respon-ses seem to make sense in describing coping with HIV/AIDS.

Coping appeared to occur in stages that roughly followed the progression from HIV infection to full-blown AIDS (Jackson, 1992). The appearance of repeated or new infections caused coping responses to change continually over time: that is, coping strategies varied over the course of a woman's illness as it became necessary to meet the needs and demands of a new situation. This makes it difficult to compare women's reports by stage of illness. Coping with HIV/AIDS is therefore not a clear process involving one major strategy, as often suggested in the literature (Lazarus, 1966; Carver, 1989). Similarly, an indivi-dual does not typically use a single coping style in dealing with HIV/AIDS. Personal tendencies and preferences for particular coping behaviours were, however, apparent. These may be related to personality characteristics, as was the case in communication about the disease.

The most remarkable observation was that all women, although supported socially, psychologically and economically by an intensive programme, largely kept silent about their HIV status. Yet self-disclosure is a prerequisite for community awareness of the threat of AIDS and to prevent further transmission. Although there were gradations in confidentiality, fear of stigma and discrimination meant that none of the women was fully open about her HIV status – even the three participants in AIDS Awareness Programmes, who told many strangers they were HIV positive. Willingness to reveal one's status did not seem to depend on marital status, economic condition, age, living conditions or education; it may be related to personality (self-efficacy, self-confidence, social competence and emotional stability). Further, as with coping, telling one's status can perhaps be seen as a process. A woman often told someone for the first time when she became ill (principally as a precaution, to have a caretaker for her children) or when there was no choice (someone suspected, or she could no longer cope economically or psychologically). The first person to whom a woman typically revealed her HIV status was her mother or sister. Many had intentions to tell a mother or sister, but they often did not succeed. Some said they could not find a way to bring up the subject or talk about it.

Rejection or abandonment by relatives or close friends, however, rarely occurred. Fear of stigmatization seemed greater than the reality. Nevertheless, three of the 19 women interviewed had experienced discrimination from relatives who suspected her of being HIV positive; this may have been enough to cause the apparently exaggerated fear of negative reactions, since these experiences were discussed in the Sikukuchwa support group. Perhaps the most striking observation was that women at Sikukuchwa even did not talk with people they met outside whom they knew or presumed to be HIV positive, although many stated they would like to help those people. It seemed clear that in Zimbabwe everyone was aware of the threat and some of the signs of HIV/AIDS (although not everyone perceived the threat to themselves), but there was a taboo on talking about it. People with HIV/AIDS looked at and suspected each other, but no one dared take the first step. Being silent has little effect, however, since people in the environment of victims often suspect or find out their HIV status. Another effect of secrecy is that people with HIV/AIDS miss emotional, social and economic support. Secrecy towards relatives, community, and even others with HIV/AIDS who do not share the secret, can result in great loneliness, thus making coping even more difficult.

HIV infection within a marital or non-marital relationship was a sensitive issue for most women. Almost none had explicitly discussed HIV with their partners, because they feared rejection and separation. Openness about the diagnosis or even suggesting the use of condoms could provoke negative reactions such as a beating, blame for being HIV positive, or abandonment. Seven of 19 relationships had broken up directly or indirectly due to HIV; of these three women were divorced and four had been deserted. Further, three experienced severe consequences after being widowed when a husband died of AIDS.[1]

At the time of the interviews five women were married and four had boyfriends. Even in marital relationships, there was hardly any discussion of HIV/AIDS. Three of the four women with boyfriends did not talk with anyone, including their boyfriends. Silence towards the partner appears to be due to the subordination (sexual or otherwise) of women in all kinds of relationships (Bassett and Mhloyi, 1991; Jackson, 1992; Berer and Ray, 1993; Meursing and Sibindi, 1995; Varkevisser, 1995); in any case it decreases possibilities for control of HIV transmission. Eight of the nine women who had a partner said they used condoms when having sexual intercourse to protect their partners and to prevent further infection for themselves. The other ten had no partner and said they preferred not to have sex. This is hardly imaginable in Zimbabwean culture, and may have been influenced by Sikukuchwa, or for some also by their age. Other women saw the problem of HIV/AIDS as a responsibility shared between them and their present partner(s). However, shared responsibility meant it was up to the partner to take action, such as deciding to use condoms. The design of strategies for women to prevent HIV infection therefore remains a difficult theme in AIDS education.

The majority of women decided they wanted no further children. Four expressed a wish for children; of these, one denied her HIV status and one was still in the process of accepting it. The other two stated they only wanted to have children if they were healthier later. Three of these four had never been married and had no children, which may have been a strong influence. In Zimbabwe, the policy is to advise HIV-positive women to avoid pregnancy: pregnant women will face disapproval from health staff and misunderstanding from the community at large. Yet women have little power to decide about condom use or family planning, so they have little control or way to protect themselves against pregnancy. Such policies on pregnancy should therefore not be carried out too rigidly.

Socioeconomic conditions in Zimbabwe had changed considerably since the time of most women's diagnosis. Meanwhile HIV/AIDS drained their resources and some potential sources of income remained underutilized due to their illness or that of a child. Separation from or desertion by a partner created even more financial consequences for seven women; those who were widowed also lost income. Most family members were not able to give economic support, and their standard of living decreased. The income-generating activities at Sikukuchwa offered them a basic income. Others who lack such support may have severe difficulty obtaining an income, so that they must turn (or return) to selling sex.

Uncertainty about the future was one of the main psychological consequences of being HIV positive. Recurring symptoms were constant reminders of their disease. Some expressed fear due to the threat to their own health, and most worried about their children's future. Since they did not talk about their HIV status with close relatives or friends, without Sikukuchwa they would have had to bear these psychological consequences almost completely on their own.

When a new woman entered Sikukuchwa, one could see that she was immediately nourished as she experienced the warmth, respect and acceptance of others in the same condition. This was often the first place women had come out with respect to their HIV status, and they experienced the help of the project as a relief. Support gave them the necessary emotional preconditions to cope with their illness. The most important function of Sikukuchwa was in giving HIV-positive women hope, and a place to talk. By encouraging and stimulating women to talk about their condition, the project supported them in managing their problems. This has also been found by Meursing, who followed HIV-positive people attending a counselling project in Bulawayo, the second largest town in Zimbabwe, over a longer span of time (Meursing, 1997).

In addition to breaking through the silence, a further role of Sikukuchwa was to provide information, care and counselling, and material support. The value of this approach was that it helped HIV-positive women – talking and working with others and playing with the children – to find individual adaptive coping strategies. They were encouraged to live positively, which meant caring for yourself and your children, eating healthy food, not thinking too much, putting trust in God and having a positive attitude towards the disease. They did not see themselves as victims and felt they could do something about their own situation. Only one woman denied her HIV status and one who had just arrived was in the process of accepting it. The rest appeared to have accepted their condition to a high degree.

According to the women, material support was very important to achieving such acceptance. They earned money from income-generating activities organized by Sikukuchwa and, if necessary, got food, clothes or money for their children's school fees or for rent. Before coming to Sikukuchwa, the situation of most was characterized by poverty and powerlessness. The project enabled and empowered HIV-positive women to care for themselves and to alter their circumstances, make plans and cope actively with their disease. That is, it gave a woman more control, or perceived control, over her own body, health and mind, and therefore her situation. Participation was also always perceived as a strong emotional help – knowledge that one is not alone and that others have even worse problems, and simple distraction. Communication with others helped women to assimilate and accept their disease, and the support group became an important source of emotional, psychological, social and practical support.

Sikukuchwa created a warm, safe and comfortable environment for coping and greatly helped HIV-positive women. On the other hand, it reduced the need for women to disclose their HIV status in their own social environment. At Sikukuchwa, the focus of coping was on the individual; the project did not consciously stimulate women to relate to others. The majority of women at Sikukuchwa discussed HIV/AIDS with each other, but did not share their problems with close relatives or talk to friends in confidence. The support of Sikukuchwa may have created an 'artificial' community, thus standing in the way of possibilities for making the community aware of people with HIV/AIDS. The self-efficacy and social competence that would have been needed to turn to those not participating at Sikukuchwa was low. Women said their reluctance was due to the lack of understanding of HIV/AIDS in the society; they perceived a low acceptance and tolerance for people with HIV/AIDS. Sikukuchwa also gave little emphasis to the possibility that women might empower themselves by collective action, which might be expected to facilitate self-disclosure both towards people with HIV/AIDS and others who do not know their HIV status. These constraints made the impact of the project less than it might have been.

Sikukuchwa received, helped and cherished HIV-positive women, but did not grow larger through them.

Though women at Sikukuchwa did not have much contact with HIV-positive women who were not participants, they expressed their concern about this large group who must face the burdens of HIV/AIDS on their own. Due to lack of time combined with ethical considerations I could not interview a control group, but some conclusions can be drawn about non-participants. Most of those interviewed complained about the scarcity of information given in hospitals or clinics when they came for testing and learned they were HIV positive. On the other hand, the women studied appeared to have a high level of knowledge. They all had a realistic concept of HIV/AIDS and gave a biomedical explanation of the cause. This knowledge had been obtained at Sikukuchwa.

Counselling in hospitals and clinics appeared incomplete or absent. Women were very unsatisfied about the amount and quality of counselling, whether pre-test (which rarely occurred) or post-test. The literature has often signalled that in the hospitals and clinics of many countries (including Zimbabwe; see e.g. Jackson, 1992), counselling is not structurally embedded in the act of informing patients about their positive status, with pre-test counselling often being ignored. A systematic, approach to both pre- and post-test counselling is a necessity. When pre-test counselling is good, patients have fewer problems in accepting a positive HIV status and in acting in ways that benefit not only themselves but also the community. Mental health care is often beyond the financial capacity of developing countries (Varkevisser, 1995). Nevertheless, the availability and quality of care and counselling, with specific attention to women's concerns, should be a central theme in HIV/AIDS control programmes. The relation and communication between health carer and patient, particularly less well-educated patients (Kleinman, 1980; Helman, 1990; van der Geest and Nijhof, 1989), as well as issues of pregnancy and motherhood (Berer and Ray, 1993) might be of particular interest.

Coming to Sikukuchwa gave women additional support and information, helping to compensate for gaps in knowledge, care and counselling. Without such a project, HIV-positive women are apt to experience all of the effects of weak support from the onset of their disease and throughout their illness: low information levels and the inviolability of counselling both have negative effects on coping with HIV/AIDS.

Women initially sought various types of healing: traditional healing (n'angas and herbalists), hospital treatment and Western medicine, and faith healing. Four women had changed their place of residence and come to Harare to obtain hospital treatment. Such a necessity for 'health' migration is a serious issue, which suggests attention to the availability of adequate treatment and counselling in rural growth points and large villages may be needed as AIDS increases everywhere and growth points attract female sex workers. Seroprevalence in these regions is still growing and cities cannot meet the increasing demand for health facilities and living space for more migrants (Bassett and Mhloyi, 1991).

Once at Sikukuchwa, the majority of women used only hospital treatment and Western medicine, although some turned to traditional treatment in times of crisis. Many in the West might consider this irrational, but for many Zimbabweans it is a logical step, as has also been documented by Cavender (1991), Bourdillon (1987), Schüssler (1992) and Farmer (1990). If one thing does not work, one tries another cure. This is also seen in Western countries, where many resort to alternative, non-conventional therapies. In this respect traditional medicine in Africa should not be seen as strange, dark, malign, or unnecessary. It might be interesting to study the impact and stimulating effects of alternative, holistic treatment on the well being of patients living with HIV/AIDS; for example traditional healers in general give more time and attention to patients than biomedical health staff.

Zimbabwe, like many other countries, found itself at an impasse. When HIV-positive people fear rejection and those in their environment fear infection, people may avoid talking to each other. The lack of education and the fear-inducing approach used in the first campaigns in Zimbabwe, stressing the incurability of HIV/AIDS and its transmission by promiscuous behaviour, seem to have been influential (Ray, 1992; Mwanga et al., 1992). Thus, though at first glance it seemed astonishing that women did not talk with others in their communities, this was not strange when one took into account the knowledge, opinions and attitudes surrounding HIV/AIDS in the society at large. Knowledge about HIV/AIDS among the general population was at least sufficient to generate intentions to change behaviour. However, knowledge and even intentions do not always translate into behavioural change (Laver, 1993; Adamchak, 1990). For women, a lack of action may often have more to do with inability than with unwillingness to change (Bassett and Mhloyi, 1991; Meursing and Sibindi, 1995). Men more often close their eyes to the risk of HIV infection or deny their HIV status (Barnett and Blaikie, 1992).

Fear of stigma caused women at Sikukuchwa to hide the cause of their suffering, and this secrecy – to which they themselves contributed – seemed to confirm the existence of severe discrimination. When a woman thinks her social environment is scared of her, laughs at her, discriminates and rejects her, she may feel the whole world is against her. Though discrimination should not be underrated, this anxiety appeared exaggerated; many may have been over-sensitive.

This perception of their communities as a threat was certainly reinforced by the existing and sometimes experienced taboos and stigma, but also may be partly explained by perceptions of who can be trusted. In the Zimbabwean socio-cultural system, the extended family is very important. Within this group of relatives there is a strong interdependence and reliance on each other. This contrasts with 'outsiders' – the wider environment, where mutual social responsibility (and therefore trust in each other) is absent. Women at Sikukuchwa seemed to put everyone outside the project in this sort of 'outsider' category, rather than being able to see individuals with different needs and opinions. Yet although people are influenced and shaped by society, probably fear HIV/AIDS and tend to reject sufferers, everyone also knows many HIV-positive persons. If this were more evident, sooner or later he or she might begin to think for themselves; people may be open enough to realize everyone – including themselves – is at risk, and that the real risk of HIV infection is not from acquaintances but from sexual practices. These HIV-positive women, however, appeared to deal with their communities as static entities that are unable to change.

In such an impasse, someone must open the discussion. On the surface, the community as a whole was not being mobilized for several reasons, including indifference, anxiety and denial. However, if one looked deeper, changes could be seen; some people were becoming curious and interested and wanted to talk about HIV/AIDS, as awareness grew that the disease affected the whole community. As Barnett and Blaikie (1992) made clear, these changes do not occur fast. Creating new concepts is time-consuming; society's coping happens in stages, and just as with individuals a society must rearrange itself. HIV/AIDS has caused profound disruption, disillusionment and disconsolation in Zimbabwean society. After initial reactions of sorrow and anger, feelings of emptiness, fear and uncertainty remain. Individuals as well as a country must face the trauma and a subsequent mourning process. HIV and AIDS must be understood and accepted by society; this is simply an acceptance of reality. The desired 'normality' described by Barnett and Blaikie (1992) will, however, take years to complete. In Zimbabwe at the time of this study, the problem had been in a sort of incubation phase for several years in which anxieties, frustration and denial had taken the upper hand. Only recently had the crisis been widely acknowledged by either government or individuals. After a period of fatalism and growing signs of stress, several initiatives for programmes for the HIV positive had emerged, and efforts were being made to control the epidemic and help the sick.

When mobilization and networking have only recently begun, revealing one's HIV status can still be a risk. As shown by the silence of women at Sikukuchwa (even those who testified in AIDS programmes) and confirmed by other researchers (Ray, 1992; Jackson, 1991; Mwanga et al., 1993; Meursing and Sibindi, 1995), there has been a tremendous taboo on talking about HIV/AIDS in Zimbabwean society. This has usually been explained as an effect of former negative AIDS prevention campaigns in the media. A few years ago, HIV-positive persons were usually advised not to tell too many people (Meursing, personal communication, 1996).

It is essential to find and develop ways to facilitate communication among women with HIV/AIDS and between these women and others. They need tools, skills and innovative ideas to help them approach people and give answers and information without indirectly and unconsciously confirming old stereotypes and prejudices. The women interviewed experienced any question a community member directed to them as an obstruction. Though not an easy task, if they could learn to take such questions seriously it could provide opportunities to talk, to explain, share, build on understanding and foster sympathy. By not answering, the women unintentionally reinforced existing stigmas and the discrimination and prejudice that flow from fear and uncertainty. Perhaps each woman participating at Sikukuchwa could be motivated and encouraged to talk with at least one woman in her daily surroundings whom she does not know but supposes to be HIV positive. To reach more women with HIV/AIDS and give them the opportunity to profit from projects like Sikukuchwa, it will be necessary to support taking such small steps.

An important objective of Sikukuchwa was to support HIV-positive women within the context of their own social environment and/or reintroduce them to normal life. Therefore a further step would be to talk with people they do not think are HIV positive. For example, as a part of efforts to avoid creating too much dependency, projects that support women with HIV and AIDS should follow a policy of encouraging women to tell their HIV status to at least one person, so that they are indeed more apt to stay in their original social context. Positive women (and men) might be stimulated to talk with close relatives and friends; their HIV status will have to be revealed to important others sooner or later in any case. Because it appeared very difficult for women at Sikukuchwa to reveal their status even to someone close to them, a first step project management might take would be to provide broader information about HIV/AIDS to close relatives/ friends and others in the women's communities, not revealing the HIV status of a particular woman. This could enable women to discuss their disease, be supported and support others. It might be useful to collect and emphasize examples of people who had successfully told others, instead of leaving women to focus on their bad experiences as those at Sikukuchwa commonly did, thereby increasing their anxiety still further.

Among the women interviewed, self-efficacy and social competence towards the social environment were low. Self-confidence and emotional stability are two qualities which projects that support women with HIV and AIDS can strengthen, mainly by making it possible for groups of women to meet in self help and support groups as at Sikukuchwa. But it is also why projects need to take the further step of seeking ways to empower women to open communications and discuss their HIV status with others. One way to do this might be to encourage women and to analyse the characteristics and skills of other women who are relatively open, and identify ways to stimulate and empower them to develop and strengthen these facilities in themselves.

At the same time, more education for the wider community is a precondition for a process that might make it possible for HIV-positive people to come out. Education in schools, beer halls, workplaces and factories was also provided by Sikukuchwa. Such education programmes may have some effect on knowledge and awareness. However, a more intensive process that, in addition to providing information, allows participants to practise communication skills and experiment with different behaviour styles as they begin to talk with relatives and friends is recommended. Further, directly confronting people with their own tendencies towards moral judgements and unintended discrimination might be more effective in HIV/AIDS prevention and in changing attitudes towards people with HIV or AIDS.

Education in Zimbabwe, as in other countries, often does not address people directly. Unfortunately, simply giving information is unlikely to change behaviour. AIDS education therefore needs more effective ways to reach both women and men, and messages designed to appeal to people and bring the personal risks of contracting HIV closer. For women, messages should make sense in relation to their subjugation to men. More people might be reached with direct emotional appeals, using messages that acknowledge the risks but do not stimulate unnecessary anxiety, give people insight into their own double standards, ambiguous and polarizing behaviour and encourage them to take personal responsibility for change. The participation of people with HIV/AIDS might facilitate this effect. A huge power could be generated by greater involvement of women like those at Sikukuchwa in AIDS education: they are young, strong and beautiful and thereby able to challenge common misconceptions and presumptions. It is necessary to stimulate discussion at all levels, so that people become familiar not only with HIV/AIDS, but also with issues of sexuality, relationships and sexual inequality, and are encouraged to make choices for themselves. This should start with discussions between men and women in communities; when the first steps have been taken, communication and acceptance may gradually become easier.

Notes

Summary

1. To maintain confidentially, Sikukuchwa is a fictitious name.

Chapter 1

1. AIDS *afflicted* households experience a direct impact: a member of the household is either ill or has died of HIV/AIDS and resources must be reallocated to deal with the problem (Barnett and Blaikie, 1992). AIDS *affected* households are affected either through the death of a family member who had contributed cash, labour or other support, or because the death or illness of a family member has meant that, for example, orphans have come to join the household.

Chapter 3

1. For many, complex diseases like HIV/AIDS are very difficult to understand. That a person can be infected but not ill, that it can take years before full-blown AIDS appears, is quite confusing. Nothing outwardly distinguishes an asymptomatic HIV-positive person from others. Yet they have a lot to think about in addition to the many difficulties of an average Zimbabwean. They should remember their status, since they can infect others, and there is a high probability they will die within a few years. People with HIV need to look after themselves carefully, and must regularly have treatment for AIDS-related diseases; often women have a baby who is repeatedly sick too.
2. The socioeconomic situation in Zimbabwe is characterized by high unemployment and poverty. Among many difficulties in Harare, the lack of social security makes life especially hard. In town everything costs money: food, accommodation – a special problem – and school. Most women expected little change in these conditions.
3. Self-efficacy is defined by Kok et al. (1987) as a person's judgement of her or his possibilities for carrying out particular behaviours. This is based on previous experience with such behaviour (in particular, attributions of success or failure), observation of others, being convinced by what others say (for example about one's skills in carrying out a particular behaviour) and physiological feedback (such as nervousness).
4. Competence relates to factors that determine whether someone has the possibilities to carry out particular behaviours, for example the degree of access to information or money and the presence or absence of skills (Wapenaar et al., 1989).
5. Traditional concepts related to the transfer of infection involve touching, sharing clothes, sharing plates or seats, and are primarily based on lack of

knowledge. Even with rational understanding, the human reaction to a frightening disease can be an emotional one. Shaking hands knowing the person is HIV positive makes people think; shaking the hand of a stranger does not evoke this reaction, even though this person could be HIV positive as well: the only difference is that the person's status is unknown.

6. According to women at Sikukuchwa, in Shona culture people talk a lot about each other. Gossip was one of their biggest fears, although they too participated. Nevertheless there was a strong taboo against talking about HIV/AIDS, so that many in the community were unaware of the disease; lack of understanding and empathy for people with HIV prevented 'telling'. Keeping silent had become a vicious circle.

Chapter 4

1. Since many people in Zimbabwe are struggling to make ends meet, when one is HIV positive, there appears to be even more reason to ask for support such as money, clothes, food or free medicine. If one wants to request such support from projects and charity organizations, being HIV positive may confer an advantage. Yet it is not impossible that some poor people with HIV who have been willing to reveal their status are better off than other poor people in Zimbabwe. Mobilization of support for people with HIV/AIDS came late, but at the time of my study many organizations in Zimbabwe were active in relation to AIDS. A paediatrician at Parirenyatwa Hospital said that, unlike many better-off patients, most poor patients are not afraid to reveal an HIV status to outsiders such as doctors, nurses, counsellors, churches and charity workers, because they know they will get something in return. Perhaps there is a relationship between poverty and opportunities to care for oneself when one is HIV positive. On the other hand, it is not possible to know whether this is a biased view.

2. Education is one of the few ways a parent can help a child to get ahead in Zimbabwe; therefore all women emphasized the need for their children to go to school. However, school expenses – uniforms, school entrance fees, money for exams – are very high. This makes it very difficult; if one does not pay the entrance fee or there is no uniform, the child will be sent home. Relatives may want to help but often can barely support themselves, let alone others. Moreover, with huge unemployment even a school diploma is no guarantee. Thus there were many reasons for women to worry about their children's future.

Chapter 6

1. It should be remembered, however, that Sikukuchwa selected participants for the relative severity of their problems.

Bibliography

Abramson P.R. and G. Herdt, 'The assessment of sexual practices relevant to the transmission of AIDS: A global perspective' , *The Journal of Sex Research*, vol. 27 (1990), pp. 215–232.

Adamchak D.J., M.T Mbizvo and M. Tawanda. 'Male knowledge of and attitudes and practices towards AIDS in Zimbabwe'. *AIDS*, vol. 4, (1990), pp. 245–250.

Barnett T. and P. Blaikie, *AIDS in Africa, its present and future impact*. London, Belhaven Press, 1992, 193 p.

Bassett T. et al., in: *Journal of Acquired Immune Deficiency Syndromes*, vol. 5, no. 6 (1992), pp. 556–559, cited in AIDS Newsletter 1992, 7(9).

Bassett M.T. and M. Mhloyi, 'Women and AIDS in Zimbabwe: the making of an epidemic'. *International Journal of Health Services*, vol. 21, no. 1 (1991), pp. 143–156.

Berer M. and S. Ray, *Women and AIDS: an international resource book*. London, Pandora Press, 1993.

Black, M., 'AIDS and Orphans in Africa. Report on a meeting'. (Meeting about AIDS and orphans in Africa, Florence, 1991.) New York, NY, UNICEF, 1991.

Bledsoe C., 'The politics of AIDS, condoms, and heterosexual relations in Africa: recent evidence from the local print media'. In: W. Penn Handweker (ed.), *Births and power. Social change and the politics of reproduction*. Boulder, Westview Press, 1990, pp. 197–223.

Bolton R., 'Rethinking anthropology: the study of AIDS'. (Unpublished paper for the conference of the AIDS Anthropology Group. University of Amsterdam, 1992.)

Bossema W., *Zimbabwe*. Koninklijk Instituut voor de Tropen (KIT)/Novib, Den Haag, SDU uitgeverij, 1990.

Bosveld W., W. Koomen and J. van der Pligt, 'False consensus: schattingen voor verschillende groepen'. In: J. van der Pligt, W. van der Kloot, A. van Knippenberg and M. Poppe (eds.) *Fundamentele sociale psychologie, deel* 5. Tilburg, Tilburg University Press, 1990.

Bourdillon M.F.C., *The Shona people*. Gweru, Mambo Press, 1987.

Bruyn, M. de, 'De risico's en gevolgen van AIDS voor vrouwen in ontwikkelingslanden'. *Medische Antropologie*, vol. 3, no. 2 (1991), pp. 236–249.

Bruyn, M. de, 'Women and AIDS in developing countries'. *Social Science and Medicine*, vol. 34, no. 3 (1992), pp. 249–262.

Bruijn, M. de, H. Jackson, M. Weijermars, V. Curtin Knight and R. Berkvens, *Facing the challenges of HIV/AIDS/STDs: a gender-based response*. Amsterdam – Royal Tropical Institute (KIT) / Harare – SAfAIDS / Geneva – World Health Organization, Global Programme on AIDS, 1995.

CADEC, 'AIDS Pilot study'. Report Catholic Development Commission. Harare. September 1991, 24 p.

Camus A., *The plague*, 1972. Quoted by R. Bolton in 'The AIDS pandemic: a global emergency'. *Medical Anthropology*, vol. 10, numbers 2–3.

Carballo M., J. Cleland, M. Carael and G. Albrecht. 'A cross national study of patterns of sexual behavior'. *The Journal of Sex Research*, vol. 26 (1989), pp. 287–299.

Carver C.S., J.K. Weintraub and M.F. Scheier 'Assessing coping strategies: a theoretically based approach'. *Journal of Personality and Social Psychology*, vol. 56, no. 2 (1989), pp. 267–283.

Cavender, A.P., 'Traditional medicine and an inclusive model of health seeking behaviour in Zimbabwe'. *Central African Journal of Medicine*, vol. 37, no. 11 (Nov. 1991), pp. 362–369.

Chibatamoto P., 'Prospective study on the criteria for diagnosis of AIDS in Zimbabwe in view of improving the reporting system in AIDS cases'. Research proposal. In: Ministry of Health and Child Welfare/National AIDS Coordination Programme, Blair Research Institute (BRI) and UNICEF (eds.), *Directory of socio-behavioural research on HIV infection and AIDS in Zimbabwe*. Harare, 1992.

Chinemana F., 'Women and HIV/AIDS in Zimbabwe: an investigation to assess needs and develop strategies'. Research protocol. In: Ministry of Health and Child Welfare/National AIDS Coordination Programme, Blair Research Institute (BRI) and UNICEF (eds.), *Directory of socio-behavioural research on HIV infection and AIDS in Zimbabwe*. Harare, 1992.

Chinemana F., G. Foster and R. Shakespeare, 'A study to investigate appropriate interventions for children orphaned as a result of AIDS in Manicaland'. Research proposal. In: Ministry of Health and Child Welfare/National AIDS Coordination Programme, Blair Research Institute (BRI) and UNICEF (eds.), *Directory of socio-behavioural research on HIV infection and AIDS in Zimbabwe*. Harare, 1992.

Conference Summary Report. *VIII International Conference on AIDS/ III STD World Congress Amsterdam*, the Netherlands 19–24 July 1992.

Dangarembga T., *Nervous conditions*. Harare, Zimbabwe Publishing House, 1990.

Darko D.F., 'A brief tour of psychoneuroimmunology'. *Annals of Allergy*, vol. 57 (1986), pp. 233–238.

Dehne C.L., 'HIV-infection in a northern district of Zimbabwe'. Abstract in Programme of the African Regional Conference of the International Epidemiological Association (IEA), August 1989, Harare.

Farmer, P., 'Sending sickness: sorcery, politics, and changing concepts of AIDS in rural Haiti'. *Medical Anthropology Quarterly*, vol. 4, no. 1 (1990), pp. 6–27.

Feldman, D.A., 'Postscript: anthropology and AIDS'. In: Feldman (ed.), *Culture and AIDS*. New York, Praeger, 1990.

Folkman S. and R.S. Lazarus, 'An analysis of coping in a middle-aged community sample'. *Journal of Health and Social Behaviour*, vol. 21 (1980), pp. 219–239.

Folkman S., M. Chesney, L. Pollack and T. Coates, 'Stress, control, coping and depressive mood in Human Immunodeficiency Virus-positive and -negative gay men in San Francisco'. *The Journal of Nervous and Mental Disease*, vol. 181 (1993) pp. 409–416.

Frank, O., 'Sexual behaviour and disease transmission in Sub-Saharan Africa: past trends and future prospects'. In Dyson (ed.), *Sexual behaviour and networking: anthropological and socio-cultural studies on the transmission of HIV*. Luijk, Derouax-Ordina, 1992, pp. 89–108.

Geest, J. van der and G. Nijhof, *Ziekte, gezondheidszorg en en cultuur. Verkenningen in de medische antropologie en sociologie*. Amsterdam, Het Spinhuis, 1989.

Gottlieb, B.H. 'Marshaling social support: the state of the art in research and practise'. In: Gottlieb (ed.), *Marshaling social support: formats, processes and effects*. Newbury Park CA., Sage, 1988, pp. 11–51.

Hampton, J., Living positively with AIDS: the AIDS support organization (TASO), Uganda.

London, ActionAid, 1991.

Hel, M. van der, 'Voorkomen is beter dan niet genezen'. *Internationale Samenwerking*, Novembre 1994, pp. 4–7.

Helman, C.G., *Culture, health and illness, an introduction for health professionals.* Oxford, Butterworth-Heinemann Ltd., 1990.

Herdt G., 'Introduction'. In: G. Herdt and S. Lindenbaum (eds.), *The time of* AIDS. London, Sage Publications Ltd., 1992, 341 p.

HIV Association Netherlands and ACT UP! Amsterdam and Bureau Women and AIDS, Utrecht, 'Report on the pre-conference women living with HIV/AIDS', 14-18 July 1992, De Born Centre, Bennekom, The Netherlands.

Hove C., *Bones.* Harare, Baobab Books, 1990.

ICWLA, 'Statement from the International Community of Women Living with AIDS'. *AIDS Health Promotion Exchange*, 1992, no. 3.

Jackson H., 'I know what I'm facing'. *Africa Health*, July (1991), pp. 30–31.

Jackson H.and K. Mambi, 'AIDS home care – a baseline survey in Zimbabwe'. V. Zimunya (ed.), *Research Series no. 3*. Harare, Journal of Social Development in Africa, School of Social Work, 1992.

Jackson H., 'AIDS: Action now. Information, prevention and support in Zimbabwe'. Harare, AIDS Counselling Trust, 1992.

Kaleeba N., 'A family commitment'. AIDS *Action* (June 1989) pp. 4–5.

Kaleeba N., S. Ray and B. Willmore, *We miss you all.* Harare, Women and AIDS Support Network (WASN) Book Project, 1991.

Katz A.H., and E.I. Bender, 'Self-help groups in western society: history and prospects'. *The Journal of Applied Behavioral Science*, vol. 12 (1976), pp. 265–282.

Kleinman, A., *Patients and healers in the context of culture.* Berkeley, University of California Press, 1980.

Kok, G.J., R.W. Meertens and H.A.M. Wilke, *Voorlichting en verandering.* Groningen, Wolters-Noordhoff, 1987.

Laver, S.M.L., 'AIDS education is more than telling people what not to do'. *Tropical Doctor*, October 1993, pp. 156–160.

Lazarus, R.S., *Psychosocial stress and the coping process.* New York, McGraw-Hill, 1966.

Lazarus, R.S. and S. Folkman, *Stress, appraisal, and coping.* New York, Springer, 1984.

Leserman J., D.O. Perkins and D.L. Evans, 'Coping with the threat of AIDS: the role of social support'. *Amercian Journal of Psychiatry*, vol. 149, no. 11 (1992), pp. 1514–1520.

Levine J., S. Warrenburg, R. Kerns, G. Schwartz, R. Delaney, A. Fontana, A. Gradman, S. Smith, S. Allen and R. Cascione, 'The role of denial in recovery from coronary heart disease'. *Psychomatic Medicine*, vol. 49 (1987), pp. 109–117.

Mann J. (1987). 'Focus on AIDS'. *WHO Features*, December 1987, pp. 9–10.

Mann J., D.J.M. Tarantola and T.W. Netter. *AIDS in the world.* Cambridge, Massachusetts, Harvard University Press, 1992, 1037 p.

Manyame B., 'Baseline survey on the need to start a home-based care project for HIV/AIDS patients'. Report Zimbabwe Red Cross Society, Harare, 1991, 26 p.

Matthews K.A., J.M. Siegel, L.H. Kuller, M. Thompson and M. Varat 'Determinants of decisions to seek medical treatment by patients with acute myocardial infarction symptoms'. *Journal of Personality and Social Psychology*, vol. 44 (1983), pp. 1144–1156.

McCombie S. C., 'AIDS in cultural, historic, and epidemiologic context'. In: Feldman
(ed.), *Culture and AIDS*, New York, Praeger, 1990.

Meursing K. and F. Sibindi, 'Coping with HIV'. *News Bulletin* vol. 2, no. 1 (1993),
Zimbabwe Women's Resource Centre & Network, Harare.

Meursing K. and F. Sibindi, *Reproductive Health Matters*, no 5 (1995), pp. 56–67.

Meursing, K., *A world of silence. Living with HIV in Matabeleland, Zimbabwe.*
Amsterdam, Royal Tropical Institute (KIT), 1997. (PhD Thesis)

Ministry of Health and Child Welfare/National AIDS Coordination Programme, Blair
Research Institute (BRI) and UNICEF (eds.), *Directory of socio-behavioural research
on HIV infection and AIDS in Zimbabwe*. Harare, 1992.

Morgan D.L., *Focus groups as qualitative research.* Beverly Hills, CA., Sage
Publications, 1988.

Murphy L.M. and A.B. Moriarty *Vulnerability, coping and growth.* New Haven and
London, Yale University Press, 1976.

Mwanga J.R., M. Dautzenberg, L.B. Chiduo, Y. Bwatwa and C. Varkevisser, 'Coping
behaviour of families with AIDS patients in Mwanza region, Tanzania'. Report
TANERA Social and Behavioral Studies, Mwanza, Tanzania, 1993.

NACP, 'Annual Report for 1991 on HIV and AIDS Surveillance', Zimbabwe, Harare, Health
information unit and National AIDS Coordination Programme, Ministry of Health and
Child Welfare, 1991.

NACP, 'HIV and AIDS Surveillance Report 1992'. Annual report, Zimbabwe, Harare,
Health information unit & National AIDS Coordination Programme, Ministry of
Health and Child Welfare, 1992.

Parker G., G. Herdt and M. Carballo, 'Sexual culture, HIV transmission, and AIDS
research'. *Journal of Sex Research*, vol. 28 (1991), pp. 77–98.

Pennebaker J.W., J.K. Kiecolt-Glaser and R. Glaser, Disclosure of traumas and immune
function: health implications for psychotherapy. *Journal of Consulting and Clinical
Psychology*, vol. 56 (1988), pp. 239–245.

Pitts M., H. Jackson and P. Wilson, 'Attitudes, knowledge, experience and behaviour
related to HIV and AIDS among Zimbabwean social workers'. *AIDS Care* vol. 2, no. 1
(1990), pp. 53–61.

Ray S. and B. Willmore, 'AIDS: an issue for every woman'. Report on the First
International Workshop on women and AIDS in Africa. Harare, Women and AIDS
Support Network, 1990.

Ray S., 'Women and AIDS Support Network: mutual support to change community
norms'. *AIDS Health Promotion Exchange*, vol. 3 (1992), pp. 4–6.

Runanga, A.O., J. Govere and Mandaza, 'The meaning of AIDS'. Research proposal. In:
Ministry of Health and Child Welfare/National AIDS Coordination Programme, Blair
Research Institute (BRI) and UNICEF (eds.), *Directory of socio-behavioural research
on HIV infection and AIDS in Zimbabwe*. Harare, 1992.

Schoepf, B.G. et al., 'AIDS, women, and society in Central Africa'. In: R. Kulstad (ed.),
AIDS 1988: *AAAS Symposia Papers*. Compact Library AIDS CD-ROM, 1988.

Schoepf, B.G., 'Political economy, sex and cultural logics: a view from Zaire'. *African
Urban Quarterly*, special issue on AIDS, HIV, STD and Urbanisation in Africa, 1992,
14 p.

Schoepf, B.G., 'The social epidemiology of women and AIDS in Africa'. In: Berer M. and
S. Ray, *Women and AIDS: an international resource book*. London, Pandora Press,
1993.

Schüssler G., 'Coping strategies and individual meanings of illness'. *Social Science and Medicine*, vol. 34, no. 4 (1992), pp. 427–432.

Sibanda T., 'Discrimination against people with HIV/AIDS and their psychological strategies of coping and adjustment'. Harare, University of Zimbabwe, Department of Psychology, 1990. (dissertation)

Spradley J.P., *The ethnographic interview*. New York, Holt, Rinehart and Winston, 1979, pp. 55–92.

Stewart M.J., 'Expanding theoretical conceptualizations of self-help groups'. *Social Science and Medicine*, vol. 31, no. 9 (1990), pp. 1057–1066.

Stichting AIDS Fonds, 'AIDS in de wereld. Kwartaaloverzicht per 15 december 1995'. *AIDS-Bestrijding*, vol. 28 (June 1996).

Stoneman C., *Zimbabwe's inheritance*. New York, St. Martin's Press, 1982.

The Herald (Zimbabwean Newspaper, 15 August 1990), *350 000–400 000 doomed to die of AIDS*.

Varkevisser C.M., I. Pathmanathan and A. Brownlee, *Designing and conducting health systems research projects. (Vol. 2) Part 1: Proposal development and fieldwork*. Health systems research (HSR) training series. Ottawa, IDRC, 1991.

Varkevisser, C.M., 'Women's health in a changing world: a continuous challenge'. *Tropical and Geographical Medicine*, vol. 47, no. 5 (1995), pp. 186–192.

VENA Journal Women and AIDS, vol. 5, no.1 (May 1993).

Wapenaar H., N.G. Röling and A.W. van den Ban, *Basisboek voorlichtingskunde*. Meppel, Boom, 1989.

World Health Organization Global Programme on AIDS, *World AIDS Day Features*, 1991, no. 4.

Willmore B. and S. Ray, 'Report of the Southern African NGO Conference on AIDS', Harare, Zimbabwe, 1990.

Woerkom, C. van, 'Massamediale voorlichting: een werkplan'. Wageningen, The Netherlands, Landbouw Universiteit, 1987.

Wolf T.M., P.M. Balson, E.V. Morse, P.M Simon, R.H Gaumer, P.W Dralle and M.H. Williams, 'Relationship of coping style to affective state and perceived social support in asymptomatic and symptomatic HIV-infected persons: implications for clinical management'. *Journal of Clinical Psychiatry*, vol. 52 (1991), pp. 171–173.

WorldAIDS, no 12 (1990) pp. 5–9 and no 13 (1991). London, Panos Institute and the Bureau of hygiene and tropical diseases.

World Bank, 'The World Bank responds to AIDS'. In: *World Bank News*, vol XIII, no. 45 (December, 1994).

Wortman C. 'Social support in cancer: conceptual and methodological issues'. *Cancer*, vol. 53 (1984), pp. 2339–2360.

Woudenberg, J.M., 'Tave kuzvigamuchira sezvazviri'. (We take it as it is). Consequences of HIV and AIDS for women in Zimbabwe, coping behaviour and support provided'. Utrecht, University of Utrecht and University of Amsterdam, 1994, 134 p. (MSc Thesis).

ANNEX 1 Important characteristics of the women

Name	Age	Marital status	Number of children	E.C.	Health status	Secrecy	Main coping strategy	Page references
Ann	23	single	2	4	HRD	3	positive reinterpretation	31, 32, 36, 40, 44, 45, 60, 61, 64, 72, 73, 75, 76, 79, 81, 83, 90, 91, 93, 94, 102, 106, 108, 109
Auxillia	39	married	3 (3 died)	5	PGL	1	acceptance	31, 43, 44, 50, 62, 73, 76, 79, 80, 90, 100
Barbara	25	widowed	3	3	HRD	2	mental disengagement	32, 33, 36, 43, 57, 63, 64, 67, 71, 72, 77, 78, 80, 87, 89, 91, 93,
Chipo	26	married	3 (1 died)	2	HRD	2	acceptance	35, 44, 53, 62, 72, 80, 81, 82, 87, 90, 94, 107, 109
Christine	23	divorced	2	3	HRD	2	planning	42, 63, 56, 65, 66, 72, 73, 76, 84, 86, 87, 106
Helen	19	boyfriend	0	3	asymp	1	denial	32, 33, 41, 45, 51, 67, 74, 79, 82, 88, 92, 101, 105, 108
Jackie	31	divorced	2 (1 died)	1	ARC	2	religion	36, 39, 42, 44, 55, 64, 67, 76, 77, 81, 90, 91, 96, 109
Joyce	29	divorced	1	1	ARC	1	religion	49, 67, 70, 76, 87, 96, 102, 108, 109, 110
Judy	26	boyfriend	2	4	PGL	1	acceptance	33, 41, 44, 50, 65, 67, 76, 79, 81, 84, 93, 94, 95, 96, 98, 99, 100, 102, 103, 105, 107, 108, 109
Marita	22	married	0 (1 died)	5	HRD	3	seeking emotional support	32, 60, 61, 64, 72, 77, 78, 88, 89, 93, 107
Noerine	31	single	0	1	HRD	1	religion	31, 42, 47, 63, 65, 75, 87, 91, 99, 103, 104, 106, 108
Nyasha	26	widowed/ boyfriend	2	4	PGL	3	seeking emotional support	31, 32, 34, 35, 39, 40, 42, 59, 61, 64, 66, 67, 71, 75, 76, 77, 79, 80, 83, 88, 89, 90, 93, 95, 96, 98, 101, 105, 107
Pretty	21	divorced/ boyfriend	1	3	asymp	1	denial	34, 50, 75, 92, 94, 104
Sarah	23	married	2	3	ARC	2	religion	31, 33, 43, 44, 54, 63, 67, 72, 73, 80, 89, 91, 96, 98, 101, 103, 105
Tambudzai	26	single	0 (1 died)	2	ARC	2	mental disengagement	57, 65, 66, 67, 74, 76, 80, 83, 87, 93, 94
Tendai	42	divorced	9 (1 died)	1	HRD	2	acceptance	31, 32, 55, 64, 66, 73, 77, 79, 80, 87, 94, 101, 105, 109

Tessa	23	married	2	5	ARC	2	seeking emotional support	31, 32, 33, 35, 40, 43, 44, 45, 54, 62, 66, 72, 74, 77, 79, 89, 92, 100, 102, 103, 104, 105, 106, 108, 109
Thandi	41	single	3 (3 died)	1	HRD	2	religion	31, 33, 36, 39, 54, 63, 64, 66, 70, 72, 81, 84, 87, 91, 95, 102, 106
Tsitsi	31	widowed	0 (1 died)	2	AIDS	1	behavioural disengagement	31, 34, 39, 41, 47, 52, 71, 80, 91, 94, 96, 97, 102, 103, 104, 106, 108

Number of children	*The first figure indicates the number of living children at the time of the interview; that in parentheses gives the number who have died*
E.C.= (economic category)	*1 = absolutely minimum income, 2 = very low income, 3 = low income, 4 = medium income relative to group, 5 = relatively higher income*
Health Status	*asymp = asymptomatic stage, PGL = Persistent Generalised Lymphadenopathy (long-lasting swollen glands), HRD = HIV Related Diseases, ARC = AIDS Related Complex, AIDS = Acquired Immune Deficiency Syndrome*
Degree of secrecy	*1= absolute secrecy, 2= selective openness, 3 = openness in AIDS Awareness Programmes*
Page references	*Pages on which quotations from the individual women can be found*

About the author

HAVERFORD COLLEGE

3 1795 00447 1833

Judith van Woudenberg began her studies in biology at the University of Utrecht, in the Netherlands, with a focus on health education and extension. Her interests, however, came to include medical anthropology, and the research among HIV-positive women in Zimbabwe on which this Bulletin is based was carried out within this framework. After graduation, Van Woudenberg was employed as a health educator at for example the STD Foundation in the Netherlands. Realizing that she wanted to work more directly and more practically with people, she began to serve as a trainer/coach. In March 1998 she began her own business, offering training and coaching in the area of career counselling and communication, including intercultural communication. Her goal is to stimulate people to uncover who they really are and what they really want in life.